Springer Series on Medical Education

Carole J. Bland, PhD, Series Editor
Steven Jones, MD, Founding Editor

Mark Quirk, EdD, is professor of family medicine and community health and has published numerous articles related to behavioral and social science research and medical education. His research has focused on faculty development, physician–patient communication, disease prevention, evaluation, cognitive development, and health education. His articles appear in journals such as *Family Medicine, Radiology, Teaching and Learning in Medicine, Social Science in Medicine, Health Psychology, Academic Medicine, International Journal of Psychology, Environment and Behavior, Preventive Medicine,* and *Merrill Palmer Quarterly.* He initiated the first required course at the University of Massachusetts Medical School (UMMS) on communication skills in 1982. He is the 2006 recipient of the STFM Excellence in Education Award, which recognizes leadership in support of teaching curriculum development and research in medical education.

Dr. Quirk has delivered invited keynote addresses on doctor–patient communication and on teaching to the Group on Educational Affairs, the International Association of Health Psychologists, and the Nordic Network for Education in Medical Communication. He has published a book on teaching and learning in medical education titled *How to Learn and Teach in Medical School.* He is an executive leader of the Macy Health Care Communication Initiative and the author of an Arthur Vining Davis Foundation Grant to develop caring attitudes among physicians.

The Clinical Faculty Development Center (CFDC) that Dr. Quirk directs has enrolled more than 800 primary care physicians from 15 medical schools in the northeastern United States. In the core program, Teaching of Tomorrow, 15 faculty members at UMMS share their educational expertise during a series of three weekend conferences each year. The CFDC also offers national workshops on medical education.

Numerous medical schools, hospitals, and professional organizations have sought consultation from Dr. Quirk in the areas of faculty development and physician communication. In addition, he has authored or coauthored successful training grants that have been funded for more than $4,000,000 since 1978. At UMMS, he is the assistant dean for academic achievement. In this role, he directs the Center for Academic Achievement (CAA), which focuses on teaching and learning in the preclinical and clinical years. Specific programs of the CAA include clinical skills electives, individual tutorials, and learning workshops for medical students, residents, and practicing physicians.

In his role as associate chair in family medicine and community health, he assists the department in academic development efforts. He chairs the Department Personnel Action Committee and is a member of the school's Basic and Clinical Science Academic Evaluation Boards and the Educational Policy Committee.

Intuition and Metacognition in Medical Education: Keys to Developing Expertise

Mark Quirk, EdD
University of Massachusetts Medical School

Foreword by John Flavell, PhD
Stanford University

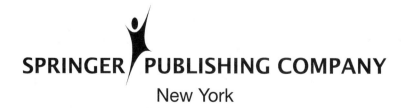

SPRINGER / PUBLISHING COMPANY
New York

Springer Publishing Company, Inc.
11 West 42nd Street
New York, NY 10036

Acquisitions Editor: Sheri W. Sussman

Managing Editor: Mary Ann McLaughlin

Production Editor: Emily Johnston

Cover design: Joanne E. Honigman

Composition: Apex Publishing

06 07 08 09 10/ 5 4 3 2 1

Library of Congress Cataloging-in-Publication Data

Quirk, Mark E.
   Intuition and metacognition in medical education : keys to developing expertise / Mark Quirk ; foreword by John Flavell.
      p. ; cm. — (Springer series on medical education)
   Includes index.
   ISBN 0–8261–0213–1
   1. Medical education. 2. Metacognition. 3. Intuition. I. Title.
II. Series: Springer series on medical education (Unnumbered)
   [DNLM: 1. Education, Medical—methods. 2. Cognition. 3. Intuition.
W 18 Q8i 2006]
R735.Q57 2006
610.71'1—dc22   2006012821

Printed in the United States of America by Bang Printing

To my father, Edward Quirk

Contents

NINE   **Teaching Expertise**

*"Teachers become expert when they . . . discover and examine
their assumptions by viewing their practice through four
distinct lenses . . . autobiographical, learners, colleagues
and literature"* —Brookfield

TEN   **Self-Directed Learning**

*"The ultimate goal is that, when school and faculty support
is no longer available, experience in clinical practice will
continue to motivate graduates, throughout their professional
careers, to use their developed skills to evaluate their performance,
identify personal learning needs, and select and evaluate
appropriate resources to achieve their goals"* —Miflin,
Campbell, and Price

ELEVEN ## A New Curricular Paradigm for Medical Education

*". . . to educate intuition it is necessary to improve the ability
to learn accurately from experience" —Hogarth*

Preface

My intended audience for this book is anyone interested in learning or teaching medicine at any point in their lives. I anticipate that a wide variety of readers, including medical school faculty, practicing physicians, students, and residents, will gain from reading these pages. It was originally a book about lifelong learning and medical education. At the time of conception, the concepts of metacognition and intuition played only supporting roles. Foresight and wisdom of the editorial board at Springer and months of reflection on the centrality of experience in learning and medical practice helped me refocus the manuscript. A judicious and lengthy review of the literature revealed that the call for lifelong learning had been initiated long ago. Despite eloquent and oft-repeated pleas for its adoption over the past century, little progress had been made. It became apparent that the reason for the widespread indifference had to do with our traditional beliefs about learning medicine.

I chose instead to focus on a new paradigm for learning in medical education that supports the development of medical expertise. Experts find answers when they don't have them. As knowledge changes, they adapt. They become *more expert* with age through experience. It became clear that our traditional paradigm for medical education was woefully outdated. In it, we not only failed to make room for continuous learning but also failed to keep up with the changing nature of learning itself. Mastery of knowledge during training, long recognized as the hallmark of expertise, would no longer serve as the foundation of *future* medical expertise. It became apparent that learning how to learn from experience and how to integrate learning and practice would accomplish this aim.

However presumptuous it was to choose to focus on a term yet to be defined in the English dictionary, the shoe seemed to fit, so to speak. Stated simply, metacognition *is* learning from experience. It is thinking about one's own or another's thoughts, feelings, and values. In specific instances, it is checking your diagnostic thinking for possible bias, seeing the illness from your patient's perspective, or reliably assessing what you need to know about a treatment option. Initially, I believed that metacognition, combined with the development of a valid and reliable knowledge base, was expertise. I didn't account for the rapid clinical decisions made by experts that often contradicted logic and led to courageous lifesaving action. It became apparent that the new paradigm for developing medical expertise must include learning from and learning to rely on one's intuition.

I am indebted to many members of the faculty at the University of Massachusetts Medical School for their support and their contributions to this book. I am particularly grateful to Angela Beeler, Frank Domino, Warren Ferguson, Melissa Fischer, Lisa Gussak, Tracy Kedian, Sarah Shields, Scott Wellman, Ilia Shlimak, Imelda Toledo-Neely, and Cheryl Killoran, who offered their narratives and ideas so that others might learn. Their expertise is truly inspirational.

I wish to thank Dan Lasser for his support as chairman and colleague. I am indebted to members of the Clinical Faculty Development Center for their willingness to join me in the intellectual pursuit of teaching teachers how to teach. Thanks to Heather-Lyn Haley for her ideas and help in mastering the literature. Special thanks to my wife Janice for her support and invaluable contribution to the ideas put forth in this book. All the clinical teachers who attended the Teaching of Tomorrow conferences and the Society of Teachers of Family Medicine Predoctoral Training Conference who offered feedback also have been instrumental in refining my ideas. Finally, the willingness of John Flavell, an eminent scholar in the field of psychology and fellow Clark University graduate, to write the foreword prompted me to reflect on my intellectual roots, for which I will always be indebted to the memory of Seymour Wapner.

Foreword

Metacognition is a very broad concept that can be roughly defined as any knowledge or cognitive activity that takes cognition as its object, or that regulates any aspect of any cognitive activity. Metacognition can include people's knowledge or intuitions about the nature of people as cognitive creatures, about the nature of different cognitive tasks, and about possible strategies for coping with different tasks. It also includes executive skills for monitoring and regulating one's cognitive activities. Acts such as self-reflection and perspective taking are clearly metacognitive in nature. The concept was introduced in the 1970s to refer to the notions about the mind that underlie children's deliberate use of memory strategies. It was subsequently extended to encompass developmental studies of cognition concerning comprehension, communication, language, perception and attention, and problem solving. During the past decade or so, there has been considerable research on metacognition in adults, and there is now even some provocative work on metacognitive-like processes in animals (sensing their own uncertainty). From the beginning, researchers have seen its potential application to learning and teaching, and there is now a considerable literature on educational applications of metacognition (for a good recent example, see Israel, Block, Bauserman, & Kinnucan-Welsch, 2005).

The present book represents an extremely interesting new educational application of the concept. In it, the author shows in fascinating detail how metacognition and intuition can be used to enhance the teaching of medical faculty and the lifelong learning of their students. The book abounds with useful, concrete suggestions for student activities that should foster metacognition and intuition as well as insightful cautions about possible overreliance on these processes.

I believe that fostering metacognition in medical teachers and students is both worth doing and feasible. It is worth doing because doctors should doctor better if they are more attuned to their own and their patients' inner states. For all the ways and reasons why this is true, I refer you to the contents of this excellent book. It should be feasible because physicians and physicians-to-be are not your everyday, run-of-the-mill learners. Rather, they are unusually intelligent individuals who have been selected for their ability to learn quickly and well. They are also highly motivated to make the right decisions because they know that patients' lives may depend on it. If really convinced that becoming more metacognitively sensitive and skilled would make them better physicians, it is hard to believe that these "superlearners" could not and would not do so. This book convinced me of its utility. I hope it will convince medical readers as well.

REFERENCE

Israel, S. E., Block, C. C., Bauserman, K. L., & Kinnucan-Welsch (Eds.). (2005). *Metacognition in literacy learning: Theory, assessment, instruction, and professional development.* Mahwah, NJ: Erlbaum.

John Flavell, PhD
Stanford University

Introduction

For more than a century, educators have exhorted curriculum leaders to adopt lifelong learning as a guiding force in medical education. Although there has been widespread agreement in principle, substantive change in this direction remains elusive. Why? Because the current paradigm for medical education does not support lifelong learning. We continue to focus the curriculum, teaching, and evaluation on the "here and now," on conveying and measuring the dissemination of current knowledge to the learner. Because of the ephemeral nature of this knowledge base, the traditional paradigm no longer prepares the physician for a lifetime of medical practice.

A new paradigm that prepares the medical student for a lifetime of learning must also prepare him or her for a lifetime of practice. The common denominator is learning from experience with patient care. The Accreditation Council of Graduate Medical Education (ACGME) has recognized the importance of this and created a separate competency called practice-based learning. The foundation for such learning begins in medical school and continues throughout the student's professional life. The preparation for lifelong practice-based learning must focus on developing the capability to regulate and monitor experience to promote future learning and continuous improvement in the quality of care. Regulating and monitoring experience is metacognition—stated simply as the ability to think about thinking and feeling. In some clinical situations, however, time limitations and complexity of the circumstances prompt the physician to rely on his or her intuition when making medical decisions. Ultimately, intuition becomes stronger through use of reflection and self-assessment, two important metacognitive capabilities.

In chapter 1, the case is made for a new paradigm for medical education that is founded on lifelong, practice-based learning. The need for change is greatly enhanced by the growing "knowledge dilemma"—there's too much, it's changing rapidly, and some is of little use. The new paradigm directs medical schools to focus on the preparation of medical experts.

Experts carefully and systematically monitor and regulate their experience but also act quickly and intuitively when necessary. Metacognition is the underlying thought process of experts that enables them to learn from experience and ultimately to act on intuition.

In chapter 2, the concept of metacognition is discussed in light of the literature on intelligence, expertise, and wisdom. Piaget, Gardner, and Flavell—familiar names in the field of psychology—were instrumental in paving the way for the development of the concept of metacognition. Their work set the stage for viewing metacognition as the thought process of experts. In this chapter, competencies of expertise are viewed as capabilities because the term more accurately depicts the ongoing nature of learning inherent in expertise. Intuition is introduced as a "partner" of metacognition in the definition of expertise.

In chapter 3, specific metacognitive capabilities for medical education are described. These capabilities can be divided into two types: regulatory strategies and strategic knowledge. Each is critical in achieving many of the other competencies defined by the ACGME (e.g., communication, professionalism, and patient care). This is accomplished through the portal of practice-based learning. Regulatory strategies are used to control thoughts and feelings. Strategic knowledge is the knowledge one has about self and how to use it. Planning and reflecting are two regulatory strategies discussed in detail. Learning style and perspective taking are two forms of strategic knowledge attended to in detail in this chapter. The risks associated with metacognition are also discussed.

Chapter 4 covers the role of intuition in medical expertise and provides a definition of its elements. The literature on the benefits of intuitive action and its impact on both learning and practice outcomes is reviewed and discussed.

In chapter 5, metacognition and intuition are portrayed as two complementary operating systems in the minds of experts. In fact, there is evidence that the development of intuition depends on metacognition. In this chapter, factors such as self-confidence, complexity, and past experience that lead the expert to choose between intuition and metacognition are discussed. This chapter will show that overuse or misuse of either intuition or metacognition can lead to medical errors, inefficiency, and distress.

Chapter 6 describes the essential roles of intuition and metacognition in medical problem solving. The elements of intuition (e.g., context dependence and pattern recognition) covered in chapter 4 and the steps of metacognition (defining the problem, mental representation, planning, and evaluation) are exemplified through clinical narratives and scripts drawn from surgery, primary care, radiology, and inpatient medicine. Characteristics of both intuition and metacognition that enhance clinical problem solving are described. These include reflecting on bias, taking the patient or family member's perspective, and recognizing patterns and subtle clues in complex situations.

Patients' perspectives are critical elements of strategic knowledge that enhance interpersonal communication. As discussed in chapter 7, self-questioning by the student or physician can be combined with direct questioning of the patient to better understand differences that influence communication in the doctor–patient relationship. It is proposed that emotional intelligence, as defined in the literature, *is* emotional metacognition. The act of apology serves as an example. The importance of first impressions (a phenomenon that grows out of intuition) and the relationship between impressions and outcomes of communication, such as patient satisfaction and stereotyping, are discussed.

Chapter 8 discusses the essential role of metacognition in the development of professionalism, a key ACGME competency area. In recent years, there has been renewed interest in professionalism as an outcome of medical education. In this chapter, a case is made for focusing the teaching of professionalism on the underlying thought processes (identity, perspective taking, reflection, and self-regulation) rather than specific behaviors (e.g., wearing a white coat or answering a page). Cultural awareness and the absence of it (e.g., stereotyping) are analyzed in terms of metacognitive capabilities. Guidance is offered for developing students' metacognitive capabilities related to several key professional attributes, including respect, honesty and integrity, and altruism.

The first eight chapters begin to define the content and goals of a curriculum devoted to achieving expertise. Chapter 9 offers specific recommendations for teaching expertise and the underlying processes of intuition and metacognition. Strategies include reflective writing and reading exercises, interactive teaching, feedback, and modeling. The reader can reflect on the value of experiential narratives, metacognitive scripts, facilitative teaching styles, and faculty self-reflections in fostering students' metacognitive skills. These strategies are brought to life with examples from colleagues and from the literature.

As described in chapter 10, metacognition depends on the student to direct much of his or her own learning. The student is required to assume greater responsibility for learning and to adapt to the learning environment. Faculty can provide students with strategies for planning (including self-assessment) and implementing learning (e.g., self-questioning and reading for comprehension). They can also introduce students to portfolios and perspective-taking techniques, such as the Review of Patient's Perspective, a critical part of the medical history.

In chapter 11, features of a curriculum that support metacognition and the development of expertise are discussed. Central to the discussion is the notion that the culture, including the values, language, rules, and aims of the medical school and medical education, must support the new paradigm. Both the formal curriculum as represented by course work and clerkships and the hidden curriculum must embrace the experiential world of the learner. The implications for student evaluation are discussed.

This book builds the case for a new paradigm that focuses on the development of medical expertise. Lifelong, practice-based learning is the key to initially achieving and, more important, maintaining competency in all areas identified by the ACGME (including patient care, medical knowledge, interpersonal communication, professionalism, and systems-based practice). Intuition and metacognition are key capabilities that underlie expertise. More studies are needed that examine the impact of metacognitive teaching and learning strategies on learning outcomes.

Intuition and Metacognition in Medical Education: Keys to Developing Expertise

CHAPTER ONE

An Emerging Paradigm for Medical Education

INTRODUCTION

In this chapter, the rationale for a new paradigm for medical education that is founded on lifelong learning is presented. It centers around the growing "knowledge dilemma" in medical education—there's too much, it is changing rapidly, and some is of little use. The new paradigm directs medical schools to focus on the preparation of medical experts as it moves toward a competency-based model. Experts carefully and systematically monitor and regulate their experience but also act quickly and intuitively when necessary. Metacognition is the underlying thought process that enables them to learn from experience and ultimately to act on their intuition.

A CASE FOR LIFELONG LEARNING

> The hardest conviction to get into the mind of a beginner is that the education upon which he is engaged is not a college course, not a medical course, but a life course, for which the work of a few years under teachers is but a preparation.
>
> *Sir William Osler (1897, p. 161)*

Osler's eloquence belies the compelling nature of his message. The rapid evolution of medical knowledge, together with an increasingly complex context of medical care, has dramatically deepened the need for a new paradigm for clinical medical education. A new approach must transform the learner's past, current, and future experience into his or her

1

ongoing "tailored" curriculum. The foundation of this personal curriculum is the ability to anticipate, plan, learn from self and others, and rapidly make clinical decisions. These abilities underlie the development of clinical expertise, an achievement that fosters perpetual self-improvement and personal quality assurance in addition to expeditious decision making in the delivery of health care.

The dizzying rate of advance in medicine challenges the traditional belief that one can prepare for a lifetime of medical practice during intensive immersion in medical school courses and residency rounds. The myth of knowledge longevity that underlies the current medical education paradigm has been evident for years. Before the turn of 20th century, the founder of *Index Medicus* lamented with reference to the published medical information he was indexing: "Nine-tenths at least [of medical information] becomes worthless and of no interest within ten years after the date of its publication" (Billings, 1887, p. 63). In fact, an astute knowledge archivist is reminded of the eminent turn-of-the-century educator Alfred North Whitehead's proclamation that "knowledge keeps no better than fish" (Whitehead, 1929, p. 98). The knowledge base has continued to expand at a torrid rate through the 21st century and has dramatically altered today's medical landscape. According to Robinson, 85% of the National Institutes of Health database is being upgraded every 5 years, available medical information is doubling every 5 years, and 90% of information learned will be obsolete in 15 years (Robinson, 1993). More than ever before, medical students must be prepared to confront the pace of advances in knowledge by continuously learning throughout their lifetimes.

Mastering the inordinate volume and ever-changing nature of knowledge required to succeed in medical practice rocks the foundation of traditional medical education. Students cannot possibly retain all of what they temporarily host for written exams and case presentations during medical school. Even the knowledge gained by those who have accurate recall for exams is extremely vulnerable to demise. Much of it becomes entrapped in the inner recesses of the mind and languishes from lack of application (Quirk, 1994). Especially vulnerable is the knowledge that goes unused for a long period of time. The solution is to be able to continuously assess and address one's learning needs as they arise and, in time-sensitive situations, rely confidently on an intuitive grasp of one's past learning experiences.

Continuous changes in the health care delivery system and growing differences in patient populations demand, more than ever, the ability to address and manage complexity. No longer can physicians view health care out of context or expect to practice medicine in a homogeneous community throughout their lifetimes. For example, they need to know how to provide care for the underserved, of which the numbers are staggering. Today, nearly 46 million Americans (16%) are uninsured (Weisman & Connolly, 2005; Kowalkzyk, 2005). Thirty-seven million Americans are living in poverty (12.7%), marking the fourth consecutive year of increases. To effectively deliver health care tomorrow, a physician will need to understand and respect the underserved patient's perspective, anticipate his or her medical needs, and advocate as well as negotiate for his or her health with a myriad of agencies. Managing complexity in clinical practice (and learning) requires the capability to understand the patient's situation, recognize one's own limitations, address individual differences, and monitor one's own thinking in action (including recognizing bias). The expert physician exercises these capabilities deliberately through metacognition or rapidly and subconsciously through intuition.

MEDICAL EXPERTISE

The movement toward competencies in medical education provides an opportunity to direct our attention to metacognitive expectations for learning. Competencies and expected learning outcomes identified by the Accreditation Council of Graduate Medical Education (ACGME), such as "communicating effectively," "using information technology," and "appraising evidence from scientific studies," must be viewed as lifetime rather than medical school achievements. The ephemeral nature of knowledge and skills, combined with the unceasing opportunities for new experiences from which to learn, expands the time frame and context for gaining competency in medicine. What is required is a learner who is competent in continuously gaining new knowledge from experience with self and others with respect to a competency area, not simply a learner who is competent in that area at any point in time. Thus, outcomes and objectives associated with a competency area should focus on the learner's current performance in that area plus his or her *capability* to continuously assess, monitor, and improve performance in that area. Defining metacognitive as well as cognitive and affective "benchmarks" for each ACGME competency can help improve performance in that area and ensure lifelong learning.

Despite the growing demands for *expert thinking* in the practice of clinical medicine, the central focus of learning in medical school courses and clerkships continues to be the development of a soon-to-be-outdated knowledge and skill base. Although important for immediate application, this approach doesn't completely prepare the student for future learning and practice. The solution is to teach learners the same skills during medical school that enable them to manage complexity in medical practice and learn throughout their lifetimes. They need to continually recognize what they know and don't know, how they best learn, how to develop and implement a plan to obtain what they need, and how to monitor their success in getting there. Specifically, medical students must develop the abilities to (a) define and prioritize their goals, (b) anticipate and assess their specific needs in relation to the goals, (c) organize (and reorganize) their experiences to meet their unique needs, (d) define their own and recognize differences in others' perspectives, and (e) continuously monitor their knowledge base, problem solving, and interactions with others.

Expertise is defined by one's capability to think as well as by the outcomes of one's thinking. Specifically, it is measured by the ability to think in a calculated and deliberate fashion and in a complementary way—by the ability to act rapidly with no apparent thought in emergent situations. As they develop their clinical expertise, medical students must learn both to think metacognitively and to act intuitively with confidence. The latter is most appropriate in response to complex problems with familiar characteristics. Some of the clinical problems they will face, however, may have new and unfamiliar characteristics, and the outcome may be much less certain. In these situations, contemplation, deliberation, and reflection are the most effective strategies. The medical school curriculum should prepare students to act deliberately or intuitively by engaging metacognitively in the learning experience.

To maximize their potential as practicing physicians and as lifelong learners, medical students must learn to effectively participate in and learn from patient care experiences throughout their productive, professional lives. They must become experts in experiential learning. They will gain knowledge from, plan for, and reflect on these experiences. It is likely that they will store what is learned in narrative form as the basis of intuition and deliberate action (Greenhalgh, 2002). Ultimately, learning from experience requires metacognition—the ability to think about one's thinking and feeling and to predict what others are thinking. Metacognition is a critical feature of the emerging paradigm for clinical learning that shifts the emphasis in medical education from application of knowledge learned in the classroom to preparing students to effectively practice medicine and learn from their experiences. It focuses on the learner's ability to regulate experience with insight about self and the ability to monitor and control knowledge rather than be overwhelmed by it.

The following two medical student–patient encounters—with the same standardized patient with the same medical complaints—illustrate the importance of metacognition in learning and medical practice. In the first encounter, Jane provides better care to the patient and learns from her experience. She seems to view the "big picture." She sees the parts in relation to the whole and understands her own and the patient's perspective in relation to the task at hand. Her ability to plan and regulate her experience leads to successful outcomes. In the second encounter, John aptly performs parts of the history and exhibits acceptable but narrowly focused problem-solving skills. For him, missed learning opportunities diminish medical and relational outcomes.

Encounter 1.1: The Metacognitive Learner

Jane, a fourth-year student, interviews Al, a patient with multiple complaints. The chart says that he is here for back pain, ringing in his ears, a bad taste in his mouth, trouble sleeping, headaches, and chest discomfort. It also notes he has missed the last three appointments. Before Jane enters the exam room, she pauses to consider her goals for the 15-minute interview. She realizes that she cannot cover the entire list of complaints and must limit and prioritize the complaints they will cover. She decides she must also address Al's chief concerns and establish a relationship with him. She recalls her tendency to overlook psychosocial issues and makes a mental note that she must elevate his three missed appointments on the problem list and not just assume that he will readily return for follow-up. She recalls previous experiences with elderly patients who had frequently missed clinic appointments because of dementia and/or depression. She will address these potential diagnoses in her history. She makes a mental note of her intuition—depression and dementia. She also realizes she needs to identify and address the barriers preventing Al from making his scheduled appointments.

One of Al's complaints is chest discomfort. Jane is confident in her knowledge and experience in this area, and she recalls an experience with an elderly patient with this complaint in her outpatient medicine rotation. That patient ultimately was diagnosed with congestive heart failure (CHF). She tells herself that this is one complaint *she must* address and decides to ask Al which of the others is most urgent from his perspective. Jane makes a mental note that she is not confident in her knowledge about another of his complaints—"ringing in the ears"—and will have to address this after the interview through some additional reading and discussion with her preceptor.

Jane knocks on the door and introduces herself to Al. She reflects to herself that Al looks much healthier and does not exhibit similar symptoms to the patient she recalled with CHF. He holds a written list of his complaints. She plans to review the list with him—perhaps this will provide further insight into his mental functioning and reveal any errors in communication that he might have had with the receptionist. After agreeing to discuss his chest discomfort, Al selects "ringing in his ears" as the complaint he would most like to resolve today. She reassesses her initial plan and will characterize the problem as best she can and make sure that she reveals her limited level of knowledge about "ringing in the ears" when she presents the patient to the preceptor. His feedback may help direct her reading on the topic.

As Al begins to describe his chest discomfort, he mentions the third-floor apartment that he lives in alone and how all his friends have either died or "gone into nursing homes." Jane reflects on what she hears in Al's words and shares his sense of loneliness. She begins to see his affect reflected in his tone and demeanor. Al then says, "I really like my apartment and get along well on my own." Jane senses that Al is concerned about having to leave his apartment and losing his independence.

Jane presents Al to the preceptor, who is impressed with her assessment, which includes depression high on the differential diagnosis list and a social service referral in her plan. Her preceptor is also impressed with the organization of her presentation, her differential, and plan.

Encounter 1.2: The Cognitive Learner

John is also a fourth-year student about to interview the same patient, Al, who presents with the same multiple complaints. John grabs the chart, knocks on the door, and introduces himself to Al, who holds a written list of his problems.

As Al looks at his list, John begins his 15-minute interview by characterizing the first problem on the patient's chart—back pain. As Al begins to describe his back pain, he mentions that he lives alone and that "all his friends have either died or gone into nursing homes." John acknowledges that it must be difficult and proceeds to question him about the "bad taste in his mouth." He does a thorough job with this and moves on to the chest discomfort. He has a great deal of knowledge in cardiovascular medicine and does a wonderful job of characterizing this problem. His 15 minutes expire before he has a chance to address any other of Al's complaints or his living situation.

After the interview, John briefly presents Al to his preceptor and ends by saying that "he did not have time to get to all of Al's complaints." He is confident in his presentation of Al's chest discomfort, and the preceptor is impressed with his recommended plan for further testing in this regard.

Both John and Jane are fourth-year students in good standing. The differences between them lie in their metacognitive capabilities. John adopts a cognitive approach to the interaction. He moves quickly through the interview in a stepwise fashion, thoroughly characterizing each complaint that he has time to cover. He did not consider the impact of the time limitation on his thought process or plan his approach. Jane, on the other hand, anticipates the limitation and creates a plan that ensures coverage of the "most serious" complaints from both her and the patient's perspective. This demonstrates an understanding of the medical consequences of the interaction and the perceived importance of the patient's perspective. She also recognizes and acts on her tendency to omit psychosocial issues from the problem list by including Al's "missed appointments."

Throughout the interview, Jane is reflective and self-monitoring, whereas John is not. She "contextualizes" her learning from previous experience by associating characteristics of this patient (i.e., elderly with missed multiple appointments) with past patients and planning to thoroughly investigate previous diagnoses. As the patient reads his complaints from the list, Jane decides that reading it together is an effective monitoring behavior that could reveal errors in communication. Based on new information—that ringing in his ears is most urgent for Al—Jane modifies her plan by including the preceptor. Finally, whereas John neglects to take the patient's perspective, Jane's capacity to do so is evident as she "shares" Al's experience of loneliness.

Both John and Jane are positively evaluated on the basis of their oral presentations to the preceptors. John's preceptor is impressed with his diagnostic knowledge and skill, particularly with chest discomfort. Jane is commended for her prioritizing, diagnostic ability, psychosocial insight, and organization. Neither preceptor, however, considers their learners' metacognitive skills and the implications for future learning and practice.

In metacognitive terms, Jane defines realistic goals, assesses what she knows and how she thinks in relation to her goals, develops a plan to achieve the goals, reflects, takes the patient's perspective, scans for errors, and modifies her plan on the basis of new information from the patient. These capabilities are generalizable and will serve her well in future learning and practice experiences. Because of these capabilities, her problem list and differential are broader and more accurate, and her plan is more appropriate. In addition, she generates a "rule" for dealing with multiple complaints and confirms that independent living can be an important "value" for some elderly patients.

Possession and use of metacognitive abilities, however, is necessary for learning but not sufficient to developing clinical expertise. The expert physician is sometimes required to act quickly without the "luxury" of conscious thinking and planning. In those situations, reliance on anticipation, planning, and reflection can result in rumination, procrastination, and accusations of perfectionism. A student who relies on metacognition in an emergency can be evaluated as inefficient, a poor decision maker, or one who lacks self-confidence or clinically doesn't get the "big picture."

Consider Roger, a fourth-year medical student who had been receiving negative evaluations by preceptors in his clerkships. Several preceptors in multiple clerkships cited his inability to act quickly as the major deficit leading to unsatisfactory performance. They stated, "He gets caught up in the minutia of cases," "He can't see the forest through the trees," "He is very unsure of himself and has difficulty making decisions," "He only wants to see a couple of patients during the morning and 'read up' on them," "He had one patient with diabetes and spent the afternoon analyzing the case and reading about the disease," and "With his experience, he should be able to do more than he does."

Roger was a very good student in the preclinical years. He possessed great insight and was rewarded for his thoughtfulness and attention to detail. However, during the "heat" of clinical medicine, he was paralyzed by his metacognitive capabilities. In this context, he was unable to "let go" of the need to reflect and could not act decisively. He became obsessive in "thinking about his thinking" and showed no intuitive capability.

Malcolm Gladwell's commentary on Goldman's algorithm for assessing acute chest pain aptly reflects Roger's challenge: "Extra information is more than useless. It's harmful. It confuses the issues. What screws up doctors when they are trying to predict heart attacks is that they take too much information into account" (Gladwell, 2005, p. 137; Goldman et al., 1996). During the premed and basic science years of his medical training, Roger had learned that *more* information was integral to clinical problem solving. He had not learned to rely on his intuition when necessary. He had not learned to balance metacognition and learning from experience with intuition and the need to act expeditiously. Advanced learners and expert clinicians alike rely on intuition when necessary and apply metacognitive capabilities as needed to learn and make clinical decisions and solve clinical problems.

METACOGNITION AS THE FOUNDATION OF LIFELONG LEARNING

In recent years, medical educators have focused on skills as the basis of curriculum reform efforts. The development of problem-based learning is representative of this shift in the cognitive arena. In a complementary fashion, reformists have also proclaimed the need to develop experiential learning abilities that extend education beyond formal training (Quirk, 1994). Echoing the words of Osler, Smith states, "The true physician never graduates from medical school; he simply transfers from Harvard, Yale, the University of California at San Francisco, or wherever medical education has been started into a new and personalized 'medical school.' In this self-created medical school, he himself will be both a faculty member and student" (Smith, 1985, p. 108). The long-established call for lifelong learning has not resulted in substantial change. This is due most likely to the absence of a suitable paradigm. Such a paradigm focuses on the attainment of medical expertise through the development of metacognitive capabilities.

Research demonstrates that learners who are strong metacognitively are more likely to achieve expertise and best prepared to learn throughout their lives. Consider one domain essential to medical expertise—reading. Metacognitively capable learners are the most effective readers because they perform *executive* functions such as budgeting and regulating reading time (Baker, 1989). In addition, they are likely to use metacognitive strategies such as visualizing, self-questioning, and reflective thinking to attain greater reading comprehension. According to Hartman, specific metacognitive reading skills that can be learned include "skimming, activating relevant prior knowledge, constructing mental images, predicting, self-questioning, comprehension monitoring, summarizing and connecting new material to prior knowledge" (Hartman, 2001, pp. 39–40). Research also suggests that medical school faculty can play an important role in facilitating students' acquisition of these metacognitive reading skills (Palincsar & Brown, 1984). In the following chapters, additional evidence is presented that contends (a) that students who are metacognitively more capable are also more effective problem solvers and communicators and (b) that metacognition can be improved through curriculum planning and teaching.

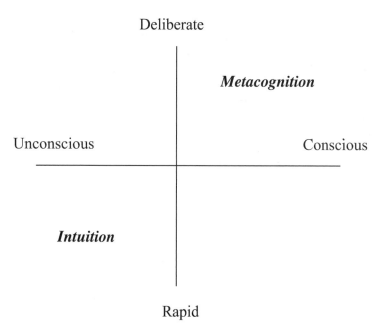

FIGURE 1.1   Clinical expertise

SUMMARY

What is proposed here is that learners systematically develop and practice metacognitive and intuitive capabilities that will serve their learning and practice needs throughout their lifetimes. Both sets of capabilities rely on learning from experience and are differentiated in practice by level of consciousness and rapidity of thinking (about thinking), as noted in Figure 1.1.

To develop intuition, it is necessary but not sufficient to practice metacognition. One must also possess self-confidence, toleration of uncertainty, and other important personal characteristics. These should be fostered in both the formal and the informal curriculum.

Clinical medical education must focus education on experience to facilitate the development of expertise. As Chauhan states, "Every life experience is a 'teachable moment'" (Chauhan, Magann, McAninch, Gherman, & Morrison, 2003, p. 203). How the lifelong learner approaches those experiences will determine the extent to which intuition and metacognition are fostered. He or she must be prepared to learn, extract the essential elements from the experience, and evaluate the results. Effective experiential learning completes the learning process. As Osler states, "To study medicine without books is like sailing in uncharted sea, but to study medicine from books alone is like never going to sea at all" (Osler, 1897, p. 161).

Research suggests that learning from experience—the foundation of clinical expertise—can be enhanced through training beyond college (Chauhan et al., 2003; Koriat & Goldsmith, 1996). As faculty, we can help learners be more vigilant about observing and interpreting their own and others' behaviors, thoughts, and feelings. Medical students, residents, and practicing physicians can develop and refine these capabilities through a lifetime of practice experience (Hernstein, Nickerson, Sanchez, & Swets, 1986; Perkins & Grotzer, 1997; Shain, 1992; Williams et al., 1996; Zimmerman, 1995).

CHAPTER TWO

Developing Expertise as the Aim of Medical Education

INTRODUCTION

This chapter describes metacognition and its place in the psychology of learning and medical education. Metacognition has become a familiar concept for research psychologists in recent decades. Both Piaget and Gardner opened the door for the concept in their writings on intelligence. Flavell coined the term in the 1970s and set the stage for viewing metacognition as the thought process of experts. In this chapter, metacognitive competencies are viewed as capabilities because the term more accurately depicts the ongoing nature of learning inherent in expertise. Intuition is identified as a "partner" of metacognition in the definition of expertise. In this chapter, several terms are introduced to frame the discussion. Table 2.1 presents definitions of these important terms to assist the reader in this chapter and subsequent ones.

There is growing consensus among educators that the aim of medical education is to develop medical expertise. The persistent popular view is that the "expert becomes so from an overwhelming mastery of content-specific knowledge" (Graber, 2003, p. 781). On the contrary, it is proposed here that the expert becomes so from an overwhelming mastery of the skills required to continuously master content-specific knowledge. This marks a fundamental shift in our approach to medical education. A more fitting definition includes the capability to continuously acquire through experience the knowledge, skills, and attitudes required to practice and learn medicine throughout a lifetime. Although content mastery is still a critical outcome, metacognition and intuition—the processes of learning

TABLE 2.1   Definitions of Essential Words

Affective	The mode of experience that relates to feelings or emotions
Benchmark	A standard of performance defined in measurable terms (Losh et al., 2005)
Capability	Extent to which individuals can adapt to change, generate new knowledge, and continue to improve their performance (Fraser & Greenhalgh, 2001)
Cognitive	The mode of experience that relates to thinking or reasoning; the process of gaining knowledge
Competence	Ability to do something well or achieve a standard
Expertise	Great knowledge and skills and the ability to control and monitor experience
Intelligence	Adaptation to the world around us; the source of action to address a need
Intuition	Knowing something without having to discover it or even be aware of it
Metacognition	Thinking about one's own or another's thinking or feeling
Problem-based learning	Educational interventions (generally small group plus independent study) that revolve around cases selected to teach aspects of clinical problem solving
Regulatory strategies	Behaviors that are used to monitor or control thoughts, feelings, or behaviors, such as checking, planning, or self-questioning
Strategic knowledge	Knowledge about one's knowledge, including how and when to use it
Wisdom	Expertise in dealing with the important and difficult aspects of life meaning and conduct (Kunzmann & Baltes, 2003)

from and acting on experience—are the capabilities of medical expertise. They are the processes by which experience is expertly transformed into medical practice and new learning over a lifetime.

INTELLIGENCE

Traditionally, the aim of any educational enterprise is the development of intelligence. Intelligence is adaptation to the world around us—the source of action to address a need. Intelligent people adapt readily, quickly, and effectively to the environment around them. In this manner, they become adept at performing their jobs and living their lives. The focus of clinical medical education is the development of intelligence required to practice clinical medicine in a complex world.

Jean Piaget, perhaps the most notable developmental psychologist of the 20th century, understood that complexity requires "higher-order" thinking and that intelligence is adaptation to that complexity (Piaget, 1972). He also surmised that the highest forms of intelligence include the ability to anticipate and reflect on our own behaviors—to think about our thoughts. He stated that "intelligence is determined by internal structures, which are likewise not formed but gradually become explicit in the course of development, owing to a reflection of thought on itself" (Piaget, 1972, p. 14). Piaget's final stage of development was defined as formal operations (or formal thought)—a stage that Piaget predicted often culminates chronologically in adolescence. The formally operating adult applies what he has learned to the process of solving new problems, implements logical strategies, and evaluates success. It is during formal thought that one is thinking about thinking, or "reflecting (in the true sense of the word) on these operations and therefore operating on operations or on their results and consequently effecting a second-degree grouping of operations" (Piaget, 1972, p. 148).

Piaget also noted that intelligence and intelligent acts include both an affective and a cognitive component. He states, "What common sense calls 'feelings' and 'intelligence,' regarding them as two opposed 'faculties,' are simply behaviour relating to persons and behaviour affecting ideas or things; but in each of these forms of behaviour, the same affective and cognitive aspects of action emerge, aspects which are in fact always associated and in no way represent independent faculties" (Piaget, 1972, p. 6). According to Piaget and many other researchers, thinking and feeling are inseparable although distinct in problem solving. Both modes of experience influence metacognitive processes such as anticipation, planning, and reflection, which are important metacognitive abilities. The timing of affective and cognitive responses in relation to these processes is unclear. There is some evidence that affective responses may precede cognitions in the problem-solving process (Zajonc, 1980). This would suggest an important role for intuition, which may actually be triggered by feelings. A new paradigm for medical education that aims at increasing clinical intelligence should focus on the development of both cognitive and affective experiential abilities.

Although Piaget laid the foundation for conceptualizing intelligence as higher-order thinking ("second-degree groupings") and as a combination of thinking and feeling, he failed to fully characterize these features. He viewed formal operations—the end point of development—as mainly cognitions about the world around us rather than as cognitions about our experience of the world around us. He did not flesh out the concept of thoughts about thoughts and feelings or thoughts about others' thoughts and feelings. Contemporary theorists and researchers working in the areas of multiple intelligences and emotional intelligence have refined thinking on these issues. They have set the stage for considering expertise as the aim of medical education and metacognition as the fundamental means of achieving this aim.

There is a growing literature on the presence of a newly identified component of intelligence that relates to emotions. Matthews, Zeidner, and Roberts (2002) have moved us closer to understanding the importance of emotion as well as cognition in explaining intelligence. Their work has implications for elevating the role of emotional intelligence as an essential ingredient of medical expertise and thus aim of medical education. Emotional intelligence may be defined as "the competence to identify and express emotions, understand emotions, assimilate emotions in thought, and regulate both positive and negative emotions in the self and in others" (Matthews et al., 2002, p. 3). This competence is evident in both "sides" of expertise—intuition and metacognition. It can be exhibited in "gut feelings" and "fight or flight" or in quiet reflections about one's own or another's feelings. Recognition and regulation of emotion *is* intelligence with implications for the physician's personal well-being, ability to care for others, and interpersonal communication skills.

The literature is quite clear that affect, specifically mood, can also "intuitively" influence decision making and performance (Ambady & Gray, 2002). One way is "mood congruency"—"the tendency to render judgments that are biased in the direction of a prevailing affective state" (Ambady & Gray, 2002, p. 947). From research, we can infer that medical students and practitioners alike who are happy, sad, depressed, anxious, or even angry may unwarily alter their clinical decision-making process. In general, research findings demonstrate that more positive mood states tend to result in more positive evaluations and vice versa (Forgas, 1998).

Howard Gardner has also expanded our understanding of intelligence and how it relates to expertise. He describes intelligence as "several relatively autonomous human competences" or as "frames of mind" (Gardner, 1983, p. 26). In Gardner's own words, he has expanded Piaget's theory of intelligence by seeking "to use the methods and overall schemes fashioned by Piaget and to focus them not merely on the linguistic, logical, and numerical symbols of classic Piagetian theory, but rather upon a full range of symbol systems encompassing musical, bodily, spatial, and even personal symbol systems" (Gardner, 1983, p. 26). He admits that the number of intelligences has not been finally identified and those that have, have not been fully described. By broadening the definition of intelligence, however, he has helped remove bias toward mathematics and deductive thinking that has infiltrated education and testing but not necessarily professional success.

In his books, Gardner painstakingly describes each of the intelligences in detail. Because they do not exist separately in reality as Gardner defines them, however, they provide little guidance to educators in the professions. In the real world, individuals' learning requirements and experiences revolve around jobs or professions that demand proficiency in many intelligences. Gardner states that combinations of skills required of the scientist, religious leader, and politician do not qualify as intelligences because they are "cultural" and "can be broken down into a collection of particular intellectual competences" (Gardner, 1983, p. 61). This would apply to the medical profession as well. There is no professional or "medical intelligence" per se that is unique. Rather, there is a set of competencies or, better yet, capabilities that range across multiple intelligences and general abilities that are critical to developing expertise in medicine or any other profession. The most effective approach to professional education is to examine the functions required and to fully describe specific capabilities related to aspects of the intelligences necessary to perform those functions.

In medicine and other professions that focus on problem solving and human relations, these capabilities would include the abilities to self-monitor and regulate performance in complex situations. As Piaget made room for *thinking about thinking* in his schema, so does Gardner in his theory of multiple intelligences. Like Piaget's "second-degree groupings" of operations, Gardner suggests that there may be a "horizontal" component that cuts across or even "oversees" the intelligences. He states that "certain more general abilities may override, or otherwise regulate, the core intelligences" (Gardner, 1983, p. 67). Self-awareness, goal directedness, information processing style, perception, and memory are among his candidates for this "higher-order thinking" component. He defines self-awareness as the "individual's exploration of his own feelings and in his emerging ability to view his own feelings and experiences in terms of the interpretive schemes and symbol systems provided by culture" (Gardner, 1983, p. 294). He also suggests the presence of an information-processing base for each intelligence related to computational capacity (e.g., phonological or grammatical for language or tonal and rhythmic for music).

Although Gardner promises to explore "empirically which connections or distinctions might obtain across" these systems, by his own admission he ultimately neglects to define and describe these "transcendent" abilities that help define intelligence (Gardner, 1983, p. 26). He is expressly unsure whether to view this set of metacognitive abilities as "a thread" that weaves through the intelligences or whether it constitutes a domain or intelligence itself.

In essence, both Piaget and Gardner set the stage for considering expertise as the aim of education, although they never fully conceptualized metacognition and its relationship to intuition. These "transcendent" abilities that they foresaw as integral to clinical problem solving and interpersonal communication (and other aspects of intelligence) are essential in the development of clinical expertise and should signify the new paradigm for medical education.

EXPERTISE

The true aim of medical education is to develop medical expertise, which embodies the higher-order thinking capabilities or "threads" alluded to by Piaget and Gardner. Experts not only have great knowledge and skills but also possess the capability to control and monitor experience. The concept of "developing expertise" captures the *dynamic* and *longitudinal* features of mastering the environment or learning from experience over one's lifetime (Sternberg, 1999). According to Sternberg, at the core of developing expertise are five elements: metacognitive skills, learning skills, thinking skills, knowledge, and motivation. The metacognitive skills defined by Sternberg include problem recognition, problem definition, problem representation, strategy formulation, resource allocation, monitoring of problem solving, and evaluation of problem solving (Sternberg, 1999).

Advancing Sternberg's approach, other researchers have begun to differentiate the novice from the expert in specific competency areas other than solving cognitive problems (Duffy, Gordon, Whelan, Cole-Kelly, & Frankel, 2004). The expert "medical communicator," for example, would rely on interpersonal expertise to elicit the patient's perspective and adjust patient education to fit the patient's needs and values. Specifically, he would recognize that the 16-year-old who reacts with concern about losing her boyfriend when told she is pregnant does not "need" to hear about her specific "options" for the pregnancy at this point in time. The expert communicator also would anticipate and recognize the emotional response by the 16-year-old and repair communication errors (such as overinforming about options rather than addressing the patient's concern about her boyfriend) "in action." In essence, the novice medical student learns to think, and the expert student learns to think about his or her thinking.

Although a significant step forward in the attempt to relate intelligence to life success through metacognition, like Piaget, Sternberg's concept of developing expertise also fails to account for rapid cognition or intuition. The learning pathway to expertise begins with generic knowledge and skills for the novice and leads to mastery of uncertainty, complexity, and decision making in new situations. This learning pathway must include metacognition as applied to experience. However, in practice (or action) experts often rely on intuition—knowing something without having to discover it or even be aware of it. In the previous example, the level of consciousness and speed with which the *recognitions* and *repairs* take place in the interaction would determine the intuitive or metacognitive nature of the responses. The features of expertise often rely on the expert's intuition or ability to rapidly assimilate and act intuitively, often triggered by feelings.

Dreyfus and Dreyfus help us understand the role of intuition in the practice of expertise. They point out that "the novice learns to recognize various objective facts and features relevant to [a new] skill and acquires rules for determining actions based upon those facts and features" (Dreyfus & Dreyfus, 1986, p. 21). The novice medical student, for example, initially operates in an environment where there are few situational or contextual contingencies to consider. He must learn the "normal heart sound" during the course in physical diagnosis by listening to a simulated demonstration on the Web and by practicing with a shiny new stethoscope on fellow students. The following semester, the student must repeat the process with "abnormal heart sounds." This student eventually becomes *competent* or *proficient* enough to apply the rules for defining the difference between heart sounds (murmurs) caused by regurgitation (valvular backflow) versus stenosis (constriction) in a 55-year-old male.

The *expert* student, resident or practitioner, on the other hand, would immediately recognize (intuit) the sound on the basis of previous or learned experience. He would "unconsciously" differentiate heart sounds to make a diagnosis without ever consciously considering the rules. In addition, he would understand that there is no "typical" abnormal heart sound, only sounds pictured in his mind as a backflow of blood through a valve versus the rush of blood through a constricted valve. He would assess situational information obtained through history, such as the patient's age, lifestyle, and family history. He would carefully observe the patient for signs and symptoms. Finally, he would reflect on his thoroughness, the accuracy of his diagnosis, and whether it "fit" his past experience. All of this would occur in less total time than it would take the "competent" learner.

CAPABILITY AND COMPETENCE

Teaching and evaluating expertise relies on the identification and evaluation of expected outcomes that are cast quite often as competencies. Competence is the ability to do something well or achieve a standard. Competencies are being defined by accrediting bodies and medical schools to represent desired outcomes of learning, and they serve widely as the basis of curriculum reform in medical education (Accreditation Council of Graduate Medical Education [ACGME], 2005). Learners are expected to demonstrate competency during medical school and residency in-patient care, medical knowledge, practice-based learning and improvement, interpersonal and communication skills, professionalism, and systems-based practice (ACGME, 2005). Ultimately, they are expected to become competent medical practitioners.

The focus on competence in medical education has beneficially elevated the role of outcomes and accountability. However, the movement toward competencies has yet to capture the full meaning of expertise. Rather than embracing the concept of continuous learning from experience throughout a lifetime, competencies have come to be viewed as static achievements (e.g., graduation from medical school, residency, fellowship, licensure, recertification, and so on). As defined by Sternberg (1999), Dreyfus and Dreyfus (1986), and other researchers, the overarching concept of expertise is dynamic, ever growing, and process oriented. It is a characteristic of interacting with and learning from the environment that one continues to refine over a lifetime. In addition, the competencies currently defined are domain specific and, like Piaget's and Gardner's schemas, fail to address the higher-order thinking capabilities of expertise that *cut across* competencies. Capability appears to be preferable to competence when defining milestones of dynamic achievement. As an outcome related to expertise, the concept of *capability*, which includes "potential," is preferred over competence because it conveys the ongoing nature of learning. Capability encompasses the "extent to which individuals can adapt to change, generate new knowledge, and continue to improve their performance" (Fraser & Greenhalgh, 2001, p. 799).

Medicine requires learners who are capable of continuously gaining new knowledge and skills from experience. The sources of new knowledge and skills are not only one's reflections on interactions with the physical and interpersonal environment around them but also one's reflections about and assessments of self and others. The "ideal physician" will possess *current* knowledge and be able to perform skills in a competency area at any point in time and also be capable of renewing this knowledge and skill base throughout his or her career.

A *benchmark* is a standard of performance defined in measurable terms (Losh et al., 2005). An example of a communication benchmark would be "by the end of the third year, the student uses common language as opposed to jargon." Through such benchmarks, capabilities can be incorporated into a spiral curriculum to address the development from novice to expert reflected in curricular goals. For example, consider the ACGME competency area "Communicate effectively and demonstrate caring and respectful behaviors when interacting with patients and their families" (ACGME, 2005). Early cognitive benchmarks of the novice first- or second-year student include behaviors such as "confirming patient identity by name" during the opening and "asking a sequence of open to closed questions when eliciting the HPI." Early affective benchmarks include behaviors such as "asking about the chief concern" and "responding with empathy to patient's losses." Metacognitive and intuitive benchmarks that signify expertise at the end of the third year of medical school include "comparing anticipated with actual patient emotional reaction to the diagnosis" and "reading patient's cues and adapting communication responses accordingly." Although these benchmark behaviors may become intuitive in practice situations, each time they are raised to the metacognitive level, new learning takes place. In this manner, attaining expertise is a lifetime achievement.

A characteristic that differentiates metacognitive from other benchmarks is that they are process oriented and provide the learner with the opportunity for further learning. Anticipating and comparing, reflecting, and taking another's perspective not only enhance the possibility of positive outcomes but also add to the experiential base for further learning. Metacognitive benchmarks can be introduced in the curriculum in each competency area to prepare the learner for and reinforce the concept of a lifelong approach to learning.

As metacognitive capabilities are achieved, the likelihood of positive outcomes is enhanced. For example, we could say that by the end of his ob/gyn clerkship, the student would be able to anticipate the concerns of a 16-year-old patient who is about to have a pelvic exam. Each time the student encounters a young patient about to have a pelvic exam, he could practice this anticipation by sharing it with his preceptor or by making a note. As the student gains more and more experience, it is expected that his anticipations will become more reliable and valid. It is a process, however, that the student will continue to develop and monitor for the remainder of his professional life. We may also expect that by the end of the clerkship the student could "reflect on his own discomfort in conducting the pelvic exam." Achieving metacognitive "benchmarks" in each competency area enhances the learner's capability to learn during related experiences (e.g., discomfort discussing HIV) and ensures lifelong learning.

Consider another example. In the ACGME-defined competency area of practice-based learning, novice students must *cognitively* be able to search the Web for the best evidence. As they progress, they must increasingly (*affectively*) feel comfortable using a PDA in the exam room to recall practice guidelines regarding use of pain medications. Finally, the expert learner must *metacognitively* reflect on his or her and others' biases and tendencies to stereotype patients who fit certain profiles, such as stereotyping as "drug seekers" young African American patients who request prescriptions for pain medication. The focus of a metacognitive capability is a mental operation rather than a feature of the environment (ACGME, 2005).

A FEW WORDS OF WISDOM

Wisdom is an essential ingredient of learning and adult adaptation—the filter that guides in selecting that which is important to know (Reeves, 1996). Medical problems do not occur in a "cognitive vacuum" and often must be solved very quickly. They have emotional and interpersonal implications for both the physician and the patient. Wisdom is evident in a physician's ability to recognize and solve problems (a) that have interpersonal features, (b) in medical situations that have great uncertainty, and or (c) where pieces of the puzzle are missing or not clearly evident.

Wisdom implies knowing from experience and relies on emotional intelligence. It "simultaneously considers and integrates the intellectual, emotional, and social underpinnings of problems as well as their implications" (Kunzmann and Baltes, 2003, p. 330). This notion that wisdom involves more than simply the cognitive domain (the traditional view of intelligence) and relies on experience makes it a most appealing term for medicine and medical problem solving.

The concept of wisdom is very similar to expertise. The wise sage knows what she knows and doesn't know, understands how she reacts emotionally, and interprets previous experience in light of new features of an uncertain situation to solve a patient's problem. These are characteristics of both medical expertise and wisdom. The wise physician possesses extraordinary intelligence about self and the field of medicine and will compassionately share her worldview with patients through empathy, education, and other means. She will likely pursue excellence with a professional demeanor in order to gain wisdom to be shared with both patients and colleagues. Expertise should include sharing with colleagues, learners, and patients alike.

The altruistic and socially just nature of wisdom is also essential to medical expertise. It is a reminder that teaching and learning expertise must include a focus on the metacognitive capabilities required for professionalism and cultural awareness. Sternberg states, "Wisdom is involved when the practical intelligence [tacit knowledge] is applied to maximizing not just one's own or someone else's self-interests, but rather a balance of various self-interests (intrapersonal) with the interests of others (interpersonal) and of other aspects of the context in which one lives (extrapersonal), such as one's city or country or environment or even God" (Sternberg, 1998, p. 354). It is truly the wise physician who considers everyone's interest, ranging from the patient to the patient's family to the health care system that we wish to cultivate (Kitchener, 1986; Kitchener & Brenner, 1990). Relying on metacognition, the solution to the problem may depend on recognizing deficits and seeking new knowledge under conditions of uncertainty, knowing from multiple perspectives (including reflecting on one's own), and committing to a decision (Reeves, 1996). To solve complex medical problems, experts often require the expansive view of multiple perspectives inherent in wisdom.

The concept of wisdom places expertise in a broader domain of life and death—often the domain of the expert physician. *Wisdom is expertise* in dealing with the important and difficult aspects of life meaning and conduct (Kunzmann & Baltes, 2003). Both are critical to patient care and professional behavior. Expert physicians share their wisdom with patients—including knowledge and skill in handling the fundamental pragmatics of life, such as life planning, life management, and life review. In sharing wisdom with others, the expert physician shares his or her sense of identity, values, and beliefs with a focus on experience.

SUMMARY

Developing expertise is the aim of medical education, and enhancing metacognitive and intuitive capabilities over a lifetime are its goals. Clinical expertise includes the ability to act intuitively—rapidly without conscious thought—in critical situations of life and death. It also requires the capability to anticipate and plan and to think about one's thinking in "new" situations. It is the latter capability that leads to new learning. This view of expertise best captures the contemporary requirements for a lifetime of medical practice—requirements that emphasize adaptation to change and management of complexity.

The two critical sets of capabilities inherent in medical expertise are metacognition and intuition. Specific metacognitive capabilities are to anticipate, plan, self-assess, reflect, and know about self and other. Specific intuitive capabilities are to feel confident with uncertainty, recognize when sufficient data have been gathered, and make decisions rapidly when necessary. Experts also wisely share the meaning they have amassed with others. This enables them to be effective teachers of patients and students.

CHAPTER THREE

Metacognitive Capabilities

INTRODUCTION

In chapter 2, a rationale for considering metacognition as a critical thought process for clinical experts was presented. The term "capability" was introduced as a more appropriate descriptor of learning outcomes than "competency" because of its focus on future as well as present learning. In this chapter, selected, specific metacognitive capabilities for medical education are discussed. Metacognitive capabilities can be divided into two types: regulatory strategies and strategic knowledge. Regulatory strategies are used to control thoughts and feelings. Strategic knowledge is the knowledge one has about self and how to use it. As competencies related to thinking and learning, each is critical in achieving other competencies such as those defined by the Accreditation Council of Graduate Medical Education (ACGME), including communication, professionalism, and patient care. Planning and reflecting are the two examples of regulatory strategies discussed in this chapter. Maximizing learning style and perspective taking are two capabilities related to strategic knowledge that are also discussed in detail. The risks associated with overusing metacognition (such as rumination) are considered here as well.

METACOGNITION

But after we have run the gamut of the simple meanings that come to one over the years, a change gradually occurs. We have grown used to the range of communication which is likely to reach us. The girl who comes to me breathless, staggering into my office, in her underwear with a still breathing infant, asking me to lock her mother out of the room; the man whose mind is gone—all of them finally saying the same thing. And then a new meaning begins to intervene. For under that language to which we have been listening all our lives a new more profound language, underlying all the dialectics offers itself. It is what they call poetry. That is the final phase.

It is that, we realize, which is beyond all they have been saying is what they have been trying to say. They laugh (For are they not laughable?); they can think of nothing more useless (What else are they but the same?); something made of words (Have they not been trying to use words all their lives?). We begin to see that the underlying meaning of all they want to tell us and have always failed to communicate is the poem, the poem which their lives are being lived to realize. No one will believe it. And it is the actual words, as we hear them spoken under all circumstances, which contain it. It is actually there, in the life before us, every minute that we are listening, a rarest element—not in our imaginations but there in fact. It is that essence which is hidden in the very words which are going in at our ears and from which we must recover underlying meaning as realistically as we recover metal out of ore. (Williams, 1984, pp. 125–126)

Medical experts possess tremendous insight into the human condition that is gained by seeing self in relation to other. Metacognition is the umbrella concept that forms the foundation of medical expertise. It is the act of *thinking about one's own and another's thinking and feeling*. In other words, the focus of this *metamental* operation is itself a mental operation (Lehrer, 1990). As the excerpt from Williams illustrates so well, metacognition is learning from experience. This can happen before an experience and take shape as anticipation, expectation, self-assessment, and planning. It can happen during or after an experience (or set of experiences) as reflection, perspective taking, and self-evaluation. The underlying assumption is that thinking is not a reflex but can be monitored and regulated deliberately because we are capable of assessing ourselves and others' reactions and directing our behaviors toward meaningful goals (Kluwe, 1982). Metacognitive capabilities can play an important role in clinical learning and practice.

The concept of metacognition has roots in the work of early-20th-century psychologists, including William James, Jean Piaget, L. S. Vygotsky, and John Dewey. It was not until the 1970s, however, that John Flavell coined the term and shaped the concept as a focus for research (Flavell, 1976, 1979). Metacognition can be defined operationally as "monitoring and management of one's thinking, including making plans before a thinking episode, regulating during the episode, and reflecting back afterwards to revise and plan future practices" (Perkins & Grotzer, 1997, p. 1128). A helpful way of thinking about metacognition is that it "reorganizes thinking by providing on-line monitoring and re-direction" (Perkins & Grotzer, 1997, p. 1128). One could argue that metacognition *is* intelligence. It is the metacognitive aspect of intelligence that enables the individual to be "not just reactive to the environment but active in forming it" (Sternberg, 1997a, p. 1030).

Medical students with strong metacognitive skills relative to those without them are going to achieve a higher level of competency as defined by the ACGME. For example, they will be more effective communicators with patients, faculty, and peers. Like many of their peers, they will demonstrate cognitive strengths, such as being able to define the content areas of a focused review of systems and the seven cardinal features of the chief complaint. They also will be able to ask an appropriate sequence of open and focused questions and summarize the history of present illness (HPI) for presentation to the preceptor. However, the developing expert who is metacognitively capable will also consider his own and the patient's experience. Specifically, he will recognize the patient's and other family members' perspectives and incorporate the patient's goals and needs into an optimal treatment and management plan. He will anticipate the patient's *chief concern* as well as potential reasons for the chief complaint. He will recognize what previous patients with similar presentations taught him and identify potential diagnoses he routinely and mistakenly omits from his differential. During the interaction, he will recognize differences between his own and the patient's perspective and redirect the interaction as the need arises to improve quality and save time. He will accurately read visual cues that tell him the patient is upset or depressed and reflect on the best way to maintain his relationship with the patient. These are the history-taking and interviewing capabilities that constitute the core curriculum of medical expertise.

So what are the metacognitive capabilities required of medical students to become expert physicians and lifelong learners? New research studies are just beginning to investigate some of these capabilities, though the unifying concept of metacognition is absent. For example, Mitchell and Liu identify three types of behaviors important for success from their interviews with medical residents: self-directed learning, critical thinking, and reflective behavior (Mitchell & Liu, 1995). In another research initiative, Gruppen is demonstrating the importance of self-assessment in medical education (Gruppen et al., 1997). As new findings emerge in these and other areas that may be related to metacognition, we must place them within a paradigm for medical education that emphasizes metacognitive as well as cognitive and affective capabilities.

A few studies now suggest that the focus in education needs to shift from teaching content to teaching learning capabilities or heuristics that include higher-order thinking (Pressley, Goodchild, Fleet, Zajchowski, & Evans, 1989). Findings in metacognition research help the way we view these capabilities. Most studies conclude that there are two broad types of metacognitive capabilities that should be taught: *regulatory strategies* (sometimes referred to as executive management strategies) and *strategic knowledge* (Hartman, 2001).

Regulatory strategies are used to monitor and control thoughts, feelings, and behaviors during a task. Specific strategies include checking, planning, selecting and goal setting, inferring, organizing, and self-questioning and self-assessing (Brown, 1978; Brown & Campione, 1977; Zimmerman, 1990). To further differentiate the nature and purpose of these strategies, Perfect and Schwartz differentiate two aspects of regulation: *monitoring* and *control* (Perfect & Schwartz, 2002). Monitoring refers to the means of achieving regulation. For example, a student studying for a physiology exam exhibits monitoring strategies when she reflects on and self-assesses her knowledge strengths and weaknesses, ease of learning, and feelings of knowing in relation to ion channels. She confidently evaluates her progress as she learns. Metacognitive control refers to the decisions one makes using the information from monitoring. For example, based on self-assessed weakness, the student plans to take the next 2 hours to study ion channels by setting objectives, choosing applicable handouts over a textbook, and allotting 1 hour for a tutorial from the appropriate faculty member. After that 3 hours, she will conduct a self-evaluation. Underlying regulatory strategies are two capabilities that will be considered in detail in this book: *reflection* and *planning*.

Strategic knowledge can be divided into three parts: *declarative*—knowledge about one's knowledge, attitudes, feelings, and skills; *contextual*—when and why to use this knowledge; and *procedural*—how to use and adapt this knowledge. Including affect as a focus of strategic knowledge broadens the implications for medical practice and learning. For example, a fourth-year student is using strategic knowledge in the clinical context when he (a) recognizes and defines his discomfort taking a sexual history, (b) decides to elicit the history with an adolescent anyway, and (c) uses strategies such as asking mom to step into the waiting room and *normalizing* the topic with the patient to reduce discomfort (for himself and the patient). Two areas of strategic knowledge that are critical to medical education are *learning style* and *others' perspectives*. Both enable the student and practicing physician alike to shape and learn from their experiences.

REGULATORY CAPABILITIES

These capabilities are employed before, during, and after an experience to enhance clinical and learning outcomes. As one educational researcher stated, "Theoreticians seem unanimous—the most effective learners are self-regulating" (Butler & Winne, 1995, p. 245). Two strategies—planning and reflection—are critical to developing medical expertise. Each of these capabilities is introduced next and discussed in greater detail in chapters 9 and 10.

Planning

Planning is a constellation of five primary monitoring and control strategies linked to the concept of continuous planning with feedback. The learner uses (a) needs assessment, anticipation, and prioritization to direct (b) objective setting and (c) method selection that in turn are used to (d) control behavior and achieve goals. Performance is evaluated (e), and the results are fed back into the process (f) (Quirk, 1994). There is ample evidence that planning is a requirement for successful learning in medicine (Candy, 1991; Quirk, 1994). One study demonstrated a positive correlation between planning behaviors and final clerkship grades, particularly the evaluation by the preceptor (Shokar, Shokar, Romero, & Bulik, 2002).

Assessing one's own needs means asking the question, What do I need to know, feel, or do according to whom? Needs must then be prioritized and considered in relation to the learning context (anticipation). Practicing self-assessment leads to positive outcomes, including skill development, academic achievement, and motivation to learn (Gordon, 1992; Westberg & Jason, 1994). There is compelling evidence that many medical students are inaccurate self-assessors, which is problematic for learning before and after graduation (Gruppen et al., 1997; Ward, Gruppen, & Regehr, 2002). This inability to self-assess grows as the stakes become higher during the third and fourth years of medical school and residency when the focus is clinical performance in such areas as problem solving and communication. In one study, Tousignant and DesMarchais (2002) found that students in the third year of a problem-based learning curriculum who completed self-assessments before and after and oral exam demonstrated poor accuracy when compared with actual performance. Another study found no relationship between medical resident self and instructor assessments in seven competency areas (Barnsley et al., 2004).

Clinical performance includes many cognitive, affective and metacognitive features that must be accounted for in the self-assessment process. If self-assessment is a more complex task when higher-order thinking and experience is involved, then one would expect less accuracy and stability in the clinical years. This is supported by Fitzgerald et al., who found that the stability of medical students' self-assessments decreased dramatically from second to third year when the focus of these assessments shifted from assessment of knowledge by written exam to assessment of clinical skills as measured by an Objective Structured Clinical Exam (OSCE) (Fitzgerald, White, & Gruppen, 2003).

Defining objectives includes identifying expected outcomes in measurable terms. This should occur during preparation for exams in the preclinical years—for example, I will be able to name the four complications of atherosclerosis—and for patient care in the clinical years—for example, I will conduct a pelvic exam and ask the mother to leave the room so that the adolescent will feel comfortable about answering questions about her sexual activity. Typically, objectives are precise, behavioral accounts that lay the groundwork for (self) evaluation. The pelvic exam and the mother leaving the room are evaluated through observation, and the patient's comfort level is best evaluated through self-report.

Once objectives are defined, the self-directed learner will choose the most appropriate methods for achieving each objective. Reading can help achieve knowledge objectives (textbooks), lead to application of knowledge (through familiarity with scripts), and also facilitate the reflective process (through narrative accounts). Using monitoring strategies such as self-questioning and visual imagery can improve comprehension at all levels. Learning methods developed early in medical school to promote cognitive learning (such as reading, note taking, storing in memory, and so on) should be complemented with clinically oriented regulatory learning methods such as self-observation and rehearsal, self-questioning, and reading narratives (e.g., with self or with preceptor) to facilitate metacognitive learning.

Weaving through needs assessment, objective setting, and method selection is the regulatory strategy of prioritization—a strategy that will impact a variety of decisions. Prioritization will focus needs assessment, such as "What aspect of diabetes treatment and management do I need to improve most?" or "What area of juvenile-onset diabetes is most challenging for me?" (Bordage & Lemieux, 1990). Prioritizing enhances the efficiency of learning (and patient care) by assigning value to needs assessment data in relation to available time and resources.

In the traditional paradigm for medical education, planning was most often considered the sole responsibility of the teacher. In the emerging paradigm, the student is featured as both learner and teacher, and planning is integral to self-directed learning. A mnemonic (GNOME) used by seasoned medical teachers to recall the five steps of planning—Goals, Needs, Objectives, Methods, Evaluation—can be adopted by learners to effectively monitor and control any learning task or activity (see chapter 10). In addition, the learner can select from a number of available instruments to assess his or her level of self-directedness (McCune, Guglielmino, & Garcia, 1990). Potential barriers to planning such as lack of organizational skills or attention difficulties can be addressed and potentially overcome through personal awareness, adoption of learning strategies, and use of technology. Planning is an essential regulatory strategy that learners must master on their way toward medical expertise.

Reflection

Learners must also simultaneously develop the capability to reflect on "ambiguity, complexity, and uncertainty" in clinical situations (Witte, 1993). Essential to both clinical practice and learning is the ability to observe and critically analyze one's own behaviors, beliefs, understanding, emotions, and attitudes in relation to the environment. In essence, reflection is learning from doing—before, during, or after the event. It can be accomplished through learning strategies such as observation and self-questioning (see chapter 10). It can be fostered by reading and writing strategies involving the narrative, the teacher's use of a facilitative teaching style, or modeling (see chapter 9).

Simply stated, reflection is observing (experiencing) while taking into account the thinking of the observer. It is linked to the attainment of important goals, such as self-awareness, self-consciousness, or self-attention (Trapnell & Campbell, 1999). Reflection is a prerequisite for effective self-assessment (reflecting on your deficits in relation to a goal). The reflective process often focuses on your interactions with other people and requires the capability of perspective taking. Consider the following illustration.

The receptionist advises the PGY III medicine resident that Mr. Jones, a patient seen in his clinic 6 months ago with mildly elevated liver function tests, is "angry, insulting, and demanding to see the doctor." He demands to know why the resident "didn't tell him he has hepatitis." Among the myriad of possible responses to the patient, the resident can (a) become angry himself and "blow the patient off," (b) justify his decision not to use the word "hepatitis," or (c) anticipate his anger, reflect on the circumstances, find out more about the patient's thoughts and feelings, and try to understand his perspective.

Being of sound metacognitive judgment, this resident chooses option c. On questioning the patient, he finds that another doctor in the emergency department reviewed the patient's chart during a recent visit for a laceration and used the word "hepatitis" to describe the previously uncovered condition. He recognizes that the patient is extremely upset when asking, "How come you never told me?" The resident sees how communication failed and accepts responsibility for the miscommunication. He apologizes and clarifies the meaning of the word "hepatitis" in relation to the previous findings.

If the resident had chosen either of the other two responses, he likely would have inflamed the situation, resulting in diminished returns. The chosen response offered the opportunity to reflect on the situation, gain strategic knowledge about the patient's perspective, and decide on an appropriate response. The capability to reflect underlies self-assessment, a skill that enhances lifelong learning and the practice of medicine (Westberg & Jason, 1994).

Reflection is a five-step process that relies on the strategy of self-questioning. To critically reflect, one must (a) account (what are the facts?), (b) assess (what is the other thinking/feeling?), (c) analyze (what are my assumptions?), (d) consider the alternatives (what could I have done instead?), and (e) define an action plan (what next?) (cf. Schön, 1987). Novack et al. advocate for reflection as a "regular part of medical training activities" and recommend that these opportunities be "integrated into existing interpersonal skills and behavioral science courses as well as clinical rotations" (Novack et al., 1997, p. 507). In chapters 9 and 10, teaching and learning strategies are offered to facilitate the development of reflection.

STRATEGIC KNOWLEDGE

Knowledge about one's cognitive strengths and weaknesses related to a clinical task and knowledge about the patient's knowledge and feelings regarding the presenting problem, diagnosis, or treatment plan constitute critical areas of strategic knowledge. Specifically, possessing and continuously updating knowledge about one's own learning style (in relation to how others learn and the task at hand) as well as knowledge about the patient gained through perspective taking are capabilities essential to medical expertise.

Learning Style

Strategic knowledge includes a practical understanding of your learning style—your cognitive strengths and weaknesses and how you learn best. Learning style is your consistent and preferred way of approaching a learning task (Curry, 1999). In a broader sense, it can include your preferred way of thinking (Sternberg, 1997b). There is an extensive literature on learning styles with varying interpretations and descriptions that include both cognitive and affective elements of learning. Although one must proceed with caution in wading through the plethora of learning-style schemata, the implications of the concept for self-understanding (metacognition) and medical education are immense (Curry, 1999).

Students' learning styles are rarely considered in developing courses of study (Davies, Rutledge, & Davies, 1995) despite the mounting evidence that style plays an important role in successful performance. In medical education, for example, there is evidence that a related concept—cognitive style—is implicated in OSCE performance and learning outcomes in the clinical context (Martin, Stark, & Jolly, 2000). In a study that involved 200 medical students, Davies et al. found that learning style was related to overall academic performance. The authors conclude that a variety of teaching methods should be available to students and that "students should be made aware of their learning styles so that they may develop better strategies to achieve success" (Davies, Rutledge, & Davies, 1995, p. 660).

There are many models available for self-assessing thinking and learning style (Dunn & Dunn, 1993; Kolb, 1984; Quirk, 1994). The one briefly summarized here is especially suited to enhance lifelong learning in medicine. It can be described along five dimensions that address the following questions: (a) How do I prefer to experience the learning material (visual, auditory, or kinesthetic)? (b) Am I more motivated to learn by exams (external) or my own interests (internal)? (c) Am I more abstract (theoretical) or concrete (step by step) in my approach to learning? (d) Do I prefer to learn from and with others or independently? and (e) Am I spontaneous or premeditated in my approach to learning? Answering these questions provides a portrait of one's learning style that can be used as strategic knowledge to plan self-directed learning experiences. Knowing one's learning style also enables one to adapt and become more flexible as the learning situations demand.

The purpose here is to orient the reader to the importance of learning style as a component of strategic knowledge rather than fully describe each of its dimensions and implications for learning. Such an undertaking would divert attention from the essential focus on metacognition. Instead, the first dimension (modes of input) will be discussed in depth to illustrate the importance of considering learning style in the new paradigm for medical education. Understanding one's personal preference for the visual, auditory, or kinesthetic mode will influence studying, help determine strengths and weaknesses, and impact on performance and career choice. Style "mismatch" can present insurmountable challenges for the ill-prepared learner. For example, if the learner prefers material in visual form, auditory learning tasks may represent a unique challenge. Identifying compensatory strategies and adapting one's learning style can significantly improve learning.

Practicing recessive dimensions of style most likely will improve performance. Practicing in "multiple dimensions" is likely beneficial for all learners. Horiszny (2001) found that exposure to heart sounds while visualizing key characteristics that physicians use to reach diagnosis leads to improved performance on an exam that involved listening to heart murmurs and identifying them. It is perhaps most important for learners with recognized limitations and will likely complement other strategies, such as rehearsal and maximizing one's preferred mode (e.g., learners who are strong visually using visual data to enhance auditory learning).

In some instances, there may be no recourse but to improve learning-style weaknesses. For example, auditory learners may need to hone visual skills to effectively read and interpret radiographs or electrocardiograms. They will compete with some visual learners who may have what Swenssen calls "search superiority" or the ability to fixate on an object in or out of context (e.g., recognize the important features such as depression of the ST segment in a cardiogram or the identifying texture and contrast of a specific lesion) (Swenssen, Hessel, & Herman, 1982). This characteristic of a strong visual style is often found in expert radiologists (Norman, Muzzin, Somers, & Rosenthal, 1992).

Students who demonstrate interest and aptitude in visually oriented specialties such as dermatology and radiology and are skilled at receiving and expressing information in images, diagrams, and charts are likely "visual learners." They will excel at tasks such as reading films and identifying rashes. Kinesthetic learners will be drawn toward "hands-on" activities such as suturing and physical examination. They will volunteer to actively participate in demonstrations and procedures. They will likely be drawn toward specialties such as surgery and orthopedics.

This dimension of learning style that is related to how we prefer to *take in* the environment around us is evident across disciplines, influences career paths, and often defines expertise. Consider how renowned architect Frank Gehry contrasts his style with the style of Esa-Pekka Salonen, the Los Angeles Philharmonic Orchestra conductor: "a musician can enter a room and sense the aural qualities the way I can sense the visual qualities" (Goldberger, 2002, p. 29). Medical students will benefit from a greater understanding of how they learn best and how they prefer to interact with the environment around them in relation to the demands of learning.

Perspective Taking

Flavell describes the "personal category" of metacognition as "thinking about cognitive differences within people, cognitive differences between people, and cognitive similarities among all people—that is, about the universal properties of human cognition" (Flavell, Miller, & Miller, 1985, p. 164). This requires perspective taking, a metacognitive capability that demands thinking about another's thoughts and feelings. Without mastery of this skill, expert communication with patients would be nonexistent. Expert perspective takers control their interpersonal interactions and relationships through mastery of empathy, patient education, and negotiation.

Learning from patients, peers, teachers, colleagues, and team members expands the learning environment and demands competence in perspective taking—the ability to seek and share in the other's view of the world. Not only will the development of this ability enhance performance in the classroom, but it will facilitate both learning and patient care in the clinic and at the bedside throughout a lifetime of medical practice.

Perspective taking develops into the ability to project oneself imaginatively into the position or situation of another. In its greatest capacity, it can evolve into a suspension of personal viewpoint so as to feel and grasp much more of the full impact of the other's experience (Fowler, 1976). It underlies our ability to develop our fund of knowledge (cognitive intelligence), emotions (emotional intelligence), and values from the world of people around us. It is a necessary prerequisite for the development of important skill sets in medicine, such as empathy (Davis, 1980, 1983), cultural sensitivity (Longhurst, 1988), negotiation in problem solving (Quirk, 1994), and professionalism (Markakis, Beckman, Suchman, & Frankel, 2000).

The ability to reliably predict, describe, and imagine the view or response of other people who may have very different experiences, concerns, and values is extremely important to learning clinical medicine. There is some evidence that medical students may not be particularly capable perspective takers. In one study, researchers examined perspective taking by having students respond to a series of case vignettes that presented problems typically encountered by students in clinical learning situations (Boenink, Oderwald, De Jong, Van Tilburg, & Smal, 2004). The situations could be analyzed from multiple perspectives, including that of the doctor, nurses, family members, patient, or societal groups. The authors found that typically the students analyzed the case from only one or two perspectives and that "hardly any weighing of perspectives took place" (Boenink et al., 2004, p. 368).

A skilled perspective taker will learn from and deliver the best care as a result of asking him- or herself the following types of questions: What is it like to be the father of a 5-year-old severely asthmatic child at midnight in the emergency room? What is it like to be a 45-year-old mother of three children who is addicted to alcohol? What is it like to try to describe your stomach pain to the nurse through an interpreter? How can I convince Mrs. Jones that her child does not need an antibiotic? They will have little difficulty negotiating and empathizing with these patients as well. Perspective taking underlies both effective care and lifelong learning in a health care system where differences and diversity are the rule rather than the exception.

Learners can develop their perspective-taking ability and learn from others by asking the right questions and analyzing the responses. On the wards, they can learn from nurses, fellow students, and residents by asking about the others' experiences with a patient. For example, often nurses will have extensive experience with the patient and can provide important insights about the patient's behavior, problems, and life.

The patient him- or herself is a valuable source of knowledge that is often untapped in a "traditional history." The review of patient's perspective can be used to complement the HPI and other important components of the history as important data-gathering strategies (see chapter 10). Residents can provide perspective to medical students that enhances patient care and the process of learning. They can provide valuable insight into their own and the attending's expectations, effective study strategies they have learned, shortcuts to save time and maintain quality in patient care, and a glimpse into the life of a learner at the next level.

For students to become effective perspective takers, faculty members must establish it as a priority in learning by including it in teaching and feedback. The patient's perspective must be a routine component of the history and expected in every student presentation.

THE RISK OF TOO MUCH METACOGNITION

There are potential risks associated with reflecting too much—particularly dwelling on potential negative outcomes of behavior. This could lead to heightened anticipatory anxiety. In fact, Wells contends that excessive metacognition is a feature of anxiety disorders (Wells, 2000). Reflecting can become rumination, or "dwelling on" potential negative outcomes that can lead to the perpetuation of negative emotions such as anxiety. Attempts to suppress the thoughts about thoughts or feelings could lead to recurrence (Wenzlaff & Wegner, 2000). This can be amplified under conditions of stress where worry and self-criticism may result from the realization that one may not be able to live up to one's unrealistic expectations (Wells, 1994). This may be particularly salient in social situations.

Matthews, Zeidner, and Roberts (2002, p. 341) refer to this aspect of metacognition as a "double-edged sword" when "decisive, problem-directed action is impeded by awareness of the private and public self." This risk is not unique to the capabilities associated with metacognition. As with other capabilities that relate to performance of the physician, "too much is not good." For example, dwelling on problem solving by generating too many hypotheses (the overextended differential diagnosis) or asking too many open questions, especially when characterizing the chief complaint (overfacilitating communication), will have a negative impact on clinical performance. These skills are not in and of themselves negative but positive. However, when used in excess or directed at inappropriate content, they most likely will lead to negative outcomes. The same will be true if one spends an inordinate amount of time overanticipating or dwelling on negative outcomes.

Learners must choose when to use and not use metacognition to enhance learning and performance. It is abundantly clear that it must be balanced by the capability to act rapidly and decisively without dwelling in thought. Ultimately, metacognition should serve intuition, its unlikely bedfellow in learning and clinical practice.

CHAPTER FOUR

The Role of Intuition

INTRODUCTION

In the first three chapters, the essential role of metacognition in expertise has been discussed. In this chapter, a case is made to include intuition in the training of medical experts. As there is a growing literature on the power of intuition, research findings from many disciplines supporting the role of intuition in expertise are discussed. It may be particularly useful for pattern recognition in complex clinical situations. Elements of intuition are presented and exemplified. The unique role of metacognition in the educational process that promotes the growth of intuition as one develops from novice to expert is introduced.

INTUITION AND OUTCOMES

Several years ago, I was working with a very competent second-year pediatric resident in my office. He presented a teenage boy who came in for a physical who also happened to have belly pain for a few days. He didn't feel it was anything serious. I specifically asked if he thought it might be appendicitis, to which he said, no. Something about the story he presented caused that small knot in my stomach that told me I need to investigate further, so I went in to see the boy. He looked fine and was only somewhat tender in his right lower quadrant. I do recall he had pain when I made him jump up and down. I really wanted to think he was fine, because he looked fine, was overall acting fine, and my competent resident thought he was fine. However, something inside me kept saying that I should be worried about him, so I made his mother take him to the emergency room. And of course, he had appendicitis. (UMMS Faculty Member, personal communication, August 21, 2005)

37

As the narrative illustrates, intuition often contravenes the reality that we observe. As this pediatrician's story suggests, acting on our intuition requires courage. A study was conducted at the University of Iowa in which people were given the task of selecting cards, one at a time, from two red and two blue decks. The red decks were "stacked" with *high* financial reward and *high* financial loss cards, whereas the cards from the blue decks provided the player with *moderate* gains and *minimal* penalties. You could win over the long run only with the blue decks. What the researchers found was that the players developed a "hunch" about what was going on by about the 50th card they selected and "figured out" that they could win only with the blue decks by about the 80th card. Gladwell summarizes the thought-to-action sequence of the players as follows: "We have some experiences. We think them through. We develop a theory. And then we finally put two and two together. That's the way learning works" (2005, p. 9).

The researchers in this study observed that the players could have followed earlier signs of intuition, resulting in even more rewarding outcomes. For example, the players had developed physiologic responses to stress (excessive sweat) when drawing from the red decks by about card 10 (Gladwell, 2005). In fact, they appeared to *unconsciously* start favoring the blue decks (taking fewer and fewer cards from the red decks) around the same time as the physiologic symptoms appeared. In essence, the players were *intuitively* responding to the experience in a maximally effective way, much earlier than they even recognized through the expression of a vague "hunch" (in fact, 400% earlier!). This leads Gladwell to conclude that some "decisions made very quickly can be every bit as good as decisions made cautiously and deliberately" (2005, p. 9).

The card experiment and the appendicitis story suggest an important role for intuition in decision making. They also suggest a special relationship between intuition and metacognition. *Following* one's intuition relies on a delicate balance between having, reflecting, and then acting on intuitive feelings. Intuitive feelings represent what has been learned though presently not articulated. In essence, intuition is based on unconscious analysis of previous experience. As Wilson (2002, p. 32) states, "Our feelings are extremely useful indicators that help us to make wise decisions. And a case can be made that the most important function of the adaptive unconscious is to generate these feelings." We might add that the most important functions of conscious behavior are to anticipate and recognize intuitive feelings, reflect on resulting actions, and plan a future course of action. This relationship between the subconscious and conscious components of learning (previous experience) marks an unlikely but essential relationship between metacognition and intuition in expertise.

It is clear that intuition can facilitate adaptation—particularly in medical situations where often the stakes are high and circumstances warrant quick action. Recent studies in clinical medicine are just beginning to demonstrate the essential role of intuition in decision making during critical situations (Crandall & Getchell-Reiter, 1993). Often these decisions entail synthesizing complicated elements from multiple experiences. As Wilson states, "The mind operates most efficiently by relegating a good deal of high-level sophisticated thinking to the unconscious, just as the modern jetliner is able to fly on automatic pilot with little or no input from the human 'conscious' pilot. The adaptive unconscious does an excellent job of sizing up the world, warning people of danger, setting goals, and initiating action in a sophisticated and efficient manner" (Gladwell, 2005, p. 12). Training medical students to generate and act confidently on intuitive feelings should be an important aim of the new paradigm in medical education. Teaching them to reflect on intuitive feelings, subsequent actions, and outcomes will enable them to learn from these experiences.

ELEMENTS OF INTUITION

Effectively practicing and teaching intuition requires an understanding of its essential elements. It is formally defined as "The state of being aware of knowing something without having to discover or perceive it" (*Dictionary*, 2005). Eminent scholar in decision making and business school leader Robin Hogarth (2001) identifies four features of intuition: (a) expertise, (b) speed of knowing, (c) lack of a deliberative thought process, and (d) experience and insight. With respect to the latter feature, he points out that there is a characteristic lack of awareness of process. Intuition in clinical medicine includes the following elements (Greenhalgh, 2002):

- Rapid, unconscious process
- Context sensitive
- Comes with practice
- Involves selective attention to small details
- Cannot be reduced to cause-and-effect logic (i.e., B happened because of A)
- Addresses, integrates, and makes sense of multiple complex pieces of data

The rapid and unconscious nature of intuition makes researching and defining it difficult. It consists of "mental processes that are inaccessible to consciousness but that influence judgments, feelings or behavior" (Wilson, 2002, p. 23). The lack of awareness that is the hallmark of intuition heightens the importance of recognizing intuitive feelings. In fact, one can question whether intuition exists at all if it isn't recognized. In this regard, intuition has been described as nothing more or less than recognition (Simon, 1992). Acting on vaguely recognized feelings when stakes are high, and observations suggest otherwise, requires acceptance of the value of intuition. Acting under these conditions requires great self-confidence (Shirlley & Langan-Fox, 1996).

A CLINICAL EXAMPLE

Intuition can be the rationale for *decisive* decision making. The ability to intuitively recognize a problem, identify a solution, or decide to act distinguishes the expert from the novice. The clinical expert "intuitively" gets the big picture and understands the relationship of the parts to the whole even if the physical "evidence" points elsewhere. In addition, the expert intuitively seems to possess an organized knowledge set for handling details during problem solving (Myers, 2002). As the following case illustrates, because intuition defies logic, even the clinical expert him- or herself often interprets it as luck:

> A 58 year old male accountant sent me an email stating the he was getting dizzy periodically. This had been going on for a week, and his wife, a nurse was pestering him to get it checked out. I called him, no chest pain, shortness of breath, no recent illness. His past history was clean: no hypertension, high cholesterol, no smoking, no family history of early heart disease, no diabetes. I brought him into the office immediately; he thought that ridiculous. His exam was completely normal. I did an EKG, and it showed he had completed a heart attack. I couldn't believe it; neither could he. I had to argue with him to go to the ER; he drove himself. He was cathed the next day, and had triple bypass 3 days later. He thinks I am a genius, I thought I was lucky. But in retrospect, I knew. I brought him in immediately, and did the EKG, because of my experience with past patients. When I thought "low risk" I was thinking disease. Now, this result goes against Bayes Theorum (a positive test result is more likely a false positive if the pre test probability is low). And 99% of the time, Bayes theorem applies. But it reminds me all the time that bad things happen, even if they are an $n = 1$ scenario. (UMMS Faculty Member, personal communication, August 13, 2005)

As Dreyfus and Dreyfus (1986, p. 108) state, "No amount of rules and facts can capture the knowledge an expert has when he has stored his experience of the actual outcomes of tens of thousands of situations." The outcomes of expert problem solving rely not on step-by-step procedures but rather on rapid correlations based on constellations of input from previous experiences. Sometimes it is one piece of data on top of all the other pieces (perhaps in the previously mentioned case it is the wife being a nurse) that sways the *intuitive decision-making process.*

INTUITION AND COMPLEXITY

Greenhalgh, a physician and medical educator, cites Sir Arthur Conan Doyle's fictitious character Sherlock Holmes as the epitome of intuition. In a response to the question of how he solved a particularly puzzling problem, Holmes states, "From long habit the train of thoughts ran so swiftly through my mind that I arrived at the conclusion without being conscious of intermediate steps" (Greenhalgh, 2002, p. 396). As one researcher, Seymour Epstein, states, "Intuition is just the things we've learned without realizing we've learned them" (in Winerman, 2005, p. 51). It is the capability to interpret experience without consciously reflecting and then to transform it into action without consciously being aware of the reasoning. The emphasis on experience as the source of action and learning leads us to include intuition as an important ingredient in expertise.

Evidence is mounting that intuition is not relegated to "lower-order" behaviors that rely on autonomic processes such as breathing, walking, or swimming. One study demonstrates the ability of intuitive power to handle complex rules for solving problems (Lewicki, Hill, & Bizot, 1988). This raises the possibility that intuition incorporates elements on metacognition at the unconscious level. The authors of this study had subjects watch a computer screen that was divided into four quadrants. Each time the screen changed, an X appeared in a different quadrant, and the subject was instructed to press a button identifying the quadrant as quickly as possible. Complex rules governed where the X would appear in each successive screen change (e.g., the third position of the X depended on the second, the fourth on the preceding two, and so on). Although subjects were able to act faster and faster in identifying the correct location as the task proceeded, they were not able to acknowledge that there was a pattern. One could make a strong argument that improvement in performance was a product of intuition. In support of this contention, when the researchers changed the operational rules, the subjects performed poorly, again without awareness of any rule change.

This is an example of where intuition—or, as Wilson refers to it, the adaptive unconscious—performs better than conscious decision making (Wilson, 2002). He notes that our intuitive or nonconscious side can perform metacognitive tasks, such as goal setting, interpretation and evaluation, and other tasks related to regulatory and executive functions.

The only difference between intuition and metacognition may be the level of consciousness in which they are employed. During intuition, metacognition may take place in the inner recesses and outside the "proper place" of consciousness (Wilson, 2002).

DEVELOPING FROM NOVICE TO EXPERT

As further testimony to the important relationship between metacognition and intuition, researchers recognize that the novice must develop his or her intuitive powers by applying metacognitive strategies. They recognize that to get to the expert stage, anticipation, deliberation, planning, and reflection are key ingredients in the learning process. Thus, honing metacognitive capabilities during medical school and residency and throughout a lifetime of clinical practice will improve *both* intuition and metacognition.

Most clinical situations encountered by the novice are new (by definition) thus ruling out an extensive experiential database that can serve as the foundation of intuitive response. The novice, then, must often act consciously—planning, anticipating, self-assessing, perspective taking, and reflecting in order to add meaning to experience. In the progression from novice to expert, it is clear that the lifelong learner will go through a number of steps that involve blending intuition and metacognition. Dreyfus and Dreyfus (1986, p. 29) define the "proficient performer," which is one step removed from the expert, as one who must still rely to a great extent on conscious application of metacognition: "The proficient performer, while intuitively organizing and understanding his task, will still find himself thinking analytically about what to do." They describe expertise as a stage for the *selected few* who treat problem solving as an extension of the many autonomic or intuitive responses that all human beings engage in every day: "We usually don't make conscious deliberate decisions when we walk, talk, drive, or carry on most social activities. An expert's skill has become so much a part of him that he need be no more aware of it than he is of his own body" (Dreyfus & Dreyfus, 1986, p. 30). Even the expert, however, must predict and anticipate novel situations and "check" intuitive decisions to avoid sloppiness, complacency, and even bias or stereotyping.

Intuition is an asset to adaptation and growth. Just as metacognitive abilities promote learning and performance, so does intuition. Both take their cues from experience. However, just as overmetacogitation can reduce efficiency, impair performance, and result in poor outcomes in certain contexts, so can the use of continuous unchecked intuition. There is evidence that intuitive judgments can be influenced and rendered less reliable by contextual factors, such as mood, previous experience, false assumptions, stereotyping, and bias (Ambady & Gray, 2002; Denes-Raj & Epstein, 1994). In the appropriate and timely context, intuitions need to be checked metacognitively. Research findings increasingly support the view that recognizing intuitive feelings and monitoring the decision-making process will lead to improved performance (Fernandez-Duque, Baird, & Posner, 2000). Wherever possible, intuitive judgments should be recognized, efficiently scrutinized, and validated in relation to observed or obtained and expected results of data gathering during the decision-making process. Dreyfus and Dreyfus (1986) state that when situational factors such as time permit, the expert will call on metacognitive capabilities. Expert decision making, they claim, does "not require calculative problem-solving, but rather involves critically reflecting on one's intuitions" (Dreyfus & Dreyfus, 1986, p. 32). In this manner, metacognition helps to ensure positive outcomes of intuitive thinking and ensure lifelong learning. Intuition is of greatest benefit to time-sensitive, spontaneous decision making. However, in the long run, using metacognition to anticipate, plan for, and reflect on behavior may mean that clinical actions will have to be repeated less often to achieve the desired results.

Perhaps the most challenging task for the novice and even the proficient learner is to decide when to rely on intuition and when to use metacognitive strategies. Learners who fail to make timely decisions and rely on intuition can be accused of being "not able to think on their feet" and "clueless." On the other hand, the "overintuitive" learner can be viewed as "sloppy" and "careless." Finding the appropriate blend of intuition and metacognition is the key to learning and ultimately to clinical expertise.

SUMMARY

Medical expertise includes the ability to make rapid, intuitive judgments and the ability to metacognitively anticipate and reflect (Bechara, Damasio, Tranel, & Damasio, 1997). In some situations, intuition or rapid metacognition will provide sufficient data about past experience to make decisions. This is particularly true in emergent situations for the expert who has great experience. The expert, however, will benefit from anticipating and recognizing intuitive feelings and reflecting on them before and after acting. Metacognition is particularly helpful to the expert in reducing medical "cognitive" errors "associated with failures in perception, failed heuristics, and biases . . . collectively referred to as cognitive dispositions to respond (CDRs)" (Croskerry, 2003, p. 775). The novice and expert alike must rely on metacognitive strategies to "check" intuition for such errors. More will be discussed about CDRs in chapter 6.

There is some evidence that intuition directs behavior at a very *general* level (i.e., pattern recognition) based on recognized similarities and differences of the current situation compared with previous experience. General physical characteristics of people and the environment can provide the basis for intuitive decision making. These generalities that lie at the intuitive level can also be responsible for stereotyping and bias, making it imperative to reflect on the decision-making process. Metacognitive strategies that check intuition for bias and stereotype are critical to the outcomes of decision making and to future learning.

Both intuition and metacognition are essential ingredients in expertise. Intuition helps physicians efficiently and effectively solve medical problems. However, it can impede performance as well. As Gladwell states, "Our unconscious reactions come out of a locked room, and we can't look inside that room. But with experience we become expert at using our behavior and our training to interpret—and decode—what lies behind our snap judgments and first impressions" (2005, p. 183). The interpretation and decoding that Gladwell refers to is metacognition.

When metacognition is applied to intuition, it is a check on the difference between the expected and the obtained outcomes and not on the differences between the obtained and the desired outcomes (Kittridge & Heywood, 2000). In essence, it is a feedback mechanism for our thinking process—a correlation between what we anticipate or predict and what we get. It is an "evaluation and adaptation of an internal model of our interaction with the world" (Kittridge & Heywood, 2000, p. 308). In addition, metacognitive reflection and planning focusing on the unique features of the current problem will address the contingencies that distinguish the current experience from previous experiences. This should enhance the probability of a positive outcome, now and in the future.

CHAPTER FIVE

Clinical Expertise: A Blend of Intuition and Metacognition

INTRODUCTION

Metacognition and intuition may be two complementary operating systems in the minds of clinical experts. Each mode of experience benefits learning and decision making, depending on the situation. In this chapter, further evidence that the development of intuition depends on metacognition is presented. Factors such as self-confidence, timing, and context that help the expert choose between intuition and metacognition are discussed. Overuse or misuse of either intuition or metacognition can lead to medical errors, inefficiency, or distress. Proceeding with caution and must be emphasized in the medical curriculum.

A COMPLEMENTARY PROCESSING SYSTEM

Intuition and metacognition are likely operating together, one at the conscious and the other at the unconscious level. Our intuitive processing system initiates the thought-to-action sequence by responding with feelings and nonconscious thoughts (based on previous experience and learning). Intuitive action can include goal setting and even evaluation of performance. Sometimes it is the *only* process we require or have time to implement. However, the novice and expert alike are often in a position to consciously and deliberately engage in planning, reflection, self-assessment, and perspective taking. These metacognitive capabilities are the foundation of lifelong learning.

Wilson proposes that "humans are blessed with two redundant systems, like modern jetliners that have backup systems in case one fails" (2002, p. 44). These systems may be less redundant than complementary. Hogarth (2001, p. 22) cites the example of a dermatologist, George, who immediately and intuitively recognizes a growth under the patient's eye because of his previous experiences. George notes that "the similarity between the growth and others of a particular type are striking." In this case, George's intuition tells him that the growth is not cancer. However, George also understands through experience that errors can be made identifying growths; therefore, it is imperative that he checks the characteristics against his knowledge base. Hogarth refers to these two processes as tacit and deliberate. They are intuition and metacognition.

These two modes of experience may share similar functions though possess distinct but supplemental features. Intuition is efficient, streamlined, and focused on the big picture. Wilson (2002) suggests different capabilities inherent in each, as represented in the approach to solving a problem. The intuitive versus the metacognitive problem solver is the pattern detector versus fact-checker, possesses a here-and-now versus the long view, and uses automatic versus controlled processing (Wilson, 2002). Medical expertise requires both sets of capabilities.

In many instances, the decision to rely on intuition or to use metacognition is the first step in the problem-solving process. One needs to ask, Is intuition sufficient in this case? Do I feel confident that there is no bias? Wilson states, "The adaptive unconsciousness is an older system designed to scan the environment quickly and detect patterns, especially ones that might pose a danger to the organism. It learns patterns easily but does not unlearn them very well; it is a fairly rigid, inflexible inference-maker" (2002, p. 66). Conscious and deliberate thought may be required. Wilson suggests that consciousness "develops more slowly and never catches up in some respects, such as the area of pattern detection. But it provides a check-and-balance to the speed and efficiency of non-conscious learning, allowing people to think about and plan more thoughtfully about the future" (p. 66). The concepts of consciousness and adaptive unconsciousness, as described by Wilson and others, provide the foundation for understanding the relationship between metacognition and intuition.

USING METACOGNITIVE CAPABILITIES TO DEVELOP INTUITION

Perhaps the most important feature of the relationship between metacognition and intuition is the inseparable nature of their development. Intuition generates experience that is the *raw material* of metacognition.

Metacognition *sharpens* subsequent clinical intuition. For example, Greenhalgh (2002, p. 399) states,

> Reflecting retrospectively on the process of clinical intuition (asking, for example, "Why did I make diagnosis X rather than diagnosis Y at that point?" Or "What prompted me to start/stop that drug?") is a powerful educational tool. In particular, critical reflection on past intuitive judgments highlights areas of ambiguity in complex decision-making, sharpens perceptual awareness, exposes the role of emotions in driving "hunches" (perhaps also demonstrating the fallibility of relying on feelings alone), encourages a holistic view of the patient's predicament, identifies specific educational needs, and may serve to "kick-start" a more analytical chain of thought on particular problems.

Dreyfus and Dreyfus (1986) also suggest that expert intuition is developed by using metacognition. They specifically implicate taking another's perspective and refer to perspective taking as a form of detached deliberation. They state, "By focusing on aspects of a situation that seem relatively unimportant when seen from one perspective, it is possible for another perspective, perhaps that of one's opponent, to spring to mind" (Dreyfus & Dreyfus, 1986, p. 38). In a patient care context, occasionally forgetting names and dates may be considered normal but is particularly worrisome for the patient whose father was recently diagnosed with Alzheimer's disease. It is not difficult to imagine that, with practice, the metacognitive capability of perspective taking becomes intuitive, or *second nature* (the patient who mentions forgetfulness is concerned about Alzheimer's). Either through intuition or metacognition, perspective taking contributes greatly to the clinical problem-solving process.

Dreyfus and Dreyfus also suggest that the ability to self-assess contributes to the intuitive side of expertise. In this regard, they propose that experts benefit from considering the "relevance and adequacy of past experiences" (1986, p. 39). In metacognitive terms, this would be referred to as self-assessment of the adequacy of prior knowledge.

INTUITION OR METACOGNITION

As an unconscious regulatory process, intuition helps the expert conserve thinking effort, thereby maintaining efficiency and sanity during the routine of everyday practice. It is an unconscious response to the routine decisions that need to be made and the behaviors that need to be implemented on a daily basis at home and at work. According to Myers (2002, p. 29), "Unconscious, intuitive inclinations detect and reflect the regularities of our personal history." These regularities may be abnormal findings in medicine. For the cardiologist, these inclinations will be generated from aberrations in data from auscultation, and for the radiologist, scanning the plain film will reveal an abnormal pattern. Intuition is also predominant in decision making when feelings may be involved. The "gut feelings" may represent a visceral response to "personality" characteristics of the patient that may even contradict the obvious. This 36-year-old with undifferentiated chest pain may actually have heart disease.

Research has demonstrated that intuition is particularly relevant in complex clinical situations that don't have an immediately visible evidence base from which to draw (Lewicki, Hill, & Czyzewska, 1992). Expert radiologists who have the ability referred to as "search superiority" rely on intuition. Intuition is also the preferred mode of experience when you don't *know that you know*. The powerful feeling you get when the mother says that her infant didn't want her bottle or when the wife (who is a nurse) thinks her husband's dizziness is serious may trigger intuition. These are instances where self-assessment is ineffective or at the very least inefficient. In these situations, it is advantageous to use intuition when decisions need to be made. As Myers (2002, p. 172) states, "In the contest between heart and head, clinicians often listen to whispers from their experiences and vote with their hearts."

In clinical decision-making situations where the potential for bias is high and the ability (and time) to gather evidence is great, deliberation and reflection should be chosen over clinical intuition. Myers (2002) cites a meta-analysis by the University of Minnesota that compared outcomes of clinical-intuitive versus mechanical-statistical predictions of behavior or prognoses. The latter was nearly eight times more accurate in predicting outcomes. As Myers states, "Clinical intuition is vulnerable to illusory correlations, hindsight biases, belief perseverance, and also to self-confirming diagnoses" (2002, p. 178). This makes clinical intuition extremely vulnerable to bias that leads to medical error. As Croskerry (2003, p. 779) states, these medical errors "lie in the shadows" and are "difficult to find." A medical school curriculum that embraces the role of intuition along with metacognition in clinical problem solving must train students to recognize the ever-present sources of bias that can impinge on the decision-making process.

Confidence can be a positive or a negative influence on intuition. Studies have shown that clinical accuracy is improved in situations when the clinician has greater confidence in his decision (McNeil, Sandberg, & Binder, 1998). Taking time to assess one's "confidence-to-knowledge" ratio will influence the choice of intuition or metacognition and enhance outcomes. However, an important caveat to remember is that people seem to be naturally overconfident. They appear to overestimate their success about 15% of the time (Brenner, Koehler, Liberman, &

Tversky, 1996; Myers, 2002). As Metcalfe (1998, pp. 100–101) states, "People think they will be able to solve problems when they won't; they are highly confident that they are on the verge of producing the correct answer when they are in fact about to produce a mistake."

Overconfidence will be difficult to detect. These types of attitudes or traits tend to rely on feelings as well as thoughts and may also be a manifestation of intuition or "unconscious memory." Wilson and Schooler (1991) posit that reflection is too analytic a process for considering reasons behind many attitudes and preferences. They state that rationalization tends to focus on the logical or plausible reasons for actions and that often the real reasons are tied to feelings or other processes that are not easily defined. Medical students should learn to accurately assess their confidence level during the decision-making process.

Simple problem-solving tasks may be more conducive to intuition than metacognition. Take, for example, simple memory tasks. Some studies have shown that "ruminating" or *overreflecting* can have a negative effect on outcomes such as visual memory (Wilson & Schooler, 1991). In an oft-quoted study on visual perception, researchers found that study participants who verbally described the faces they saw relative to participants who did not were less likely to recognize those faces again (Schooler & Engstler-Schooler, 1990).

Research suggests that rumination or "priming" with negative thoughts can also lead to negative outcomes. Even when the intention is to control for the negative thoughts, attentional load and distraction can "force" the unwanted behavior to occur (Wegner, 1994). The irony is that the unwanted behavior is more likely to occur than if no attempt to control it is implemented. This implies that in certain emergency situations where fear or panic may be prevalent, it is best to not attempt to control an unwanted action or feeling by reflecting but to simply *go with one's instincts*.

On the other hand, those same instincts that form the basis of intuition—first impressions derived from previous experience—may also prove wrong. Once again, visual perception provides a worthy example. Myers (2002, p. 1) states, "My geographical intuition tells me that Reno is east of Los Angeles, that Rome is south of New York, that Atlanta is east of Detroit. But I am wrong, wrong, wrong." Studies have demonstrated that reliance on intuition in these situations will negatively affect problem solving. In another study, most participants were influenced by visual perception and decided against logic. They chose to blindly draw a red jelly bean from a flat bowl of 100 that contained between 5 and 9 red out of 100 white (clearly stated as 5% to 9% chance rather than a bowl of 10 that contained 9 white and 1 red (clearly stated 10% chance) (Denes-Raj & Epstein, 1994). It is interesting to note that the researchers found an association between study outcomes and real-life behavior related to gambling.

Not only can intuition based on false perception lead us down the wrong path in solving problems or answering everyday questions, it can negatively influence interpersonal perceptions as well. In this regard, studies support the nonconscious influence of perceived physical characteristics on human behavior. For example, Gladwell's (2005) informal study of Fortune 500 companies showed that height is positively associated with being a chief executive officer (CEO) of a major company (nearly 6 feet to an average of 5 feet 9 inches in the general population). He states that 14.5% of the U.S. population is 6 feet or taller—58% of Fortune 500 CEOs are. In addition, 3.9% of men are 6 feet 2 inches or taller—nearly one-third of his CEOs are. These findings support the findings of other studies that show a relationship between height and success (Judge & Cable, 2004).

Unchecked intuition can also lead to significant "maladaptive" social behavior (Winerman, 2005). In this regard, there is evidence that intuitive or unconscious responses are the basis of negative stereotypes such as racism and age discrimination (Bargh, Chen, & Burrows, 1996). For example, intuition can be influenced by general differences in appearance or the color of one's skin or the shape of one's face. Results of the *Implicit Association Test* provide evidence of these potential biases and stereotyping that result from "thin slicing" or first impressions that underlie intuition (Greenwald, McGhee, & Schwartz, 1998; Lewicki et al., 1992). Repeated administrations of that test show that when "positive" terms are paired with African American photos, subjects take much more time to recognize (on a conscious level) the terms as positive relative to when these same photos are paired with negative terms to be recognized.

Some studies demonstrate the shortcomings of intuition related to visual perception in medicine. Researchers found that, with other historical, physical examination, demographic, and even personality factors controlled, standardized patients of different racial and gender backgrounds who presented with chest pain were treated differently (Shulman et al., 1999). Whites and males relative to blacks and females were referred for cardiac catheterization significantly more often even when physicians' beliefs about the probabilities of coronary artery disease were controlled. These authors suggest that the physicians' behaviors may be the result of subconscious perceptions rather than overt prejudice because of the absence of a logical connection between their explicit problem solving (overall assessment of the patient with respect to the presence of coronary artery disease) and their ultimate referral behavior. They state, "Subconscious bias occurs when a patient's membership in a target group automatically activates a cultural stereotype in the physician's memory regardless of the level of prejudice the physician has" (p. 625).

SUMMARY

Intuition can play a major positive role in medical expertise. It is a powerful ally in clinical decision-making situations constrained by time where solutions rely on immediate pattern recognition and there is a lack of accessible evidence or undue complexity. It allows the expert to "leap into action" when necessary and when all the pieces to the puzzle are not evident or available. Intuition embraces emotion and rapid cognition, requires self-confidence, and relies on pattern recognition to solve problems. These features that prove advantageous in some circumstances, however, can be disadvantageous in others. Intuition is vulnerable to bias and stereotyping, and the recognized patterns may overshadow contextual details that differentiate a given situation from the routine.

CHAPTER SIX

Clinical Problem Solving

INTRODUCTION

The first five chapters provide a rationale for defining a new paradigm for medical education that fosters the development of expertise through metacognition. The critical role of intuition in learning and practice, as well as its relationship to metacognition, has been discussed. Chapter 6 focuses the discussion on clinical problem solving, an essential element of patient care (a competency of the Accreditation Council of Graduate Medical Education). The elements of intuition (e.g., context dependence and pattern recognition) defined in chapter 4 and the steps of metacognition (defining the problem, mental representation, planning, and evaluation) are exemplified through clinical narratives and scripts that focus on the clinical problem-solving process. The examples are drawn from surgery, primary care, radiology, and inpatient medicine. Characteristics of both intuition and metacognition that enhance clinical problem solving are described. These include reflecting on bias, taking the patient or family member's perspective, and recognizing patterns and subtle clues in complex situations.

THE ROLE OF INTUITION IN THE NEONATAL INTENSIVE CARE UNIT

I have been working in the NICU for over 20 years. Infants' conditions change so rapidly that it does take some experience to recognize the subtle clues. This 3-week-old, 30-weeker was doing well. She was off oxygen, in an isolette (incubator), and doing some bottle-feeding. The baby's mother came to visit and hold the baby every day.

When I came to work at 7:00 P.M., the baby's mother was holding her. I asked her how she was doing, and she stated that the baby was quiet today and didn't really take her bottle by mouth. The day nurse said that they had done a bath with the baby and that maybe it tired her out. She was placed back into her isolette at 8:00 P.M. The baby was due for a feeding and an assessment at 9:00 P.M. The baby's temperature was low normal. I had to increase the isolette temperature. She was also a little mottled. She was having some apnea and bradycardia (heart rate drop) that had increased over the day. (UMass Memorial Healthcare nurse, personal communication)

The nurse's intuition "told her" to pay particular attention to this infant. As she explains, "When I teach newer NICU staff, I tell them that infants can change very quickly. They have to pay attention to even the smallest changes in the infant. It is important to listen to the mother describe changes in the infant's behavior. Sometimes you have a feeling about the infant. They don't look quite right. They are not very reactive to handling; maybe just a little pale or mottled."

Within a few hours' time of heightened awareness and after careful monitoring, a sepsis work-up was done with this infant, and antibiotics were started. The infant had the start of necrotizing endocolitis that was caught in time. After a week of antibiotics and feedings on hold, the infant was able to restart feeds slowly and ultimately did well. Intuition—or the "ability to pay attention to even the smallest changes in infants"—is crucial to patient care in the NICU. With reference to her highly vulnerable and dependent neonates, the nurse states, "An infection could kill them in a very short period of time. I have seen that happen and when I feel a baby 'isn't quite right.' I have to be my patients' advocate because they can't speak for themselves."

There is a growing literature describing the importance of intuition in *expert* clinical problem solving that solidifies its place in the emerging paradigm for medical education (Abernathy & Hamm, 1995). In the real world, expert clinicians often employ intuitive capabilities along with logico-deductive reasoning and evidence-based medicine to solve pressing medical problems. NICU nurses often treat sepsis intuitively *and appropriately* with antibiotics when it would not be warranted by traditional tests (Crandall & Getchell-Reiter, 1993). As in the previously cited narrative, expert nurses often act on vaguely described cues related to patterns of infant behavior that are not well documented in the literature. In one study, the authors reach a plausible conclusion that the NICU nurses use intuition (pattern recognition) to make rapid clinical decisions with little "clinical data" (Crandall & Getchell-Reiter, 1993). They suggest that their expertise allows them to rely on their intuition to recognize even the most subtle cues and variations in the patterns of behavior exhibited by infants (e.g., changes in responsiveness or color) in these critical cases.

In many respects, intuition is reliance on clinical experience to modify the findings of evidence-based medicine. Crandall and Getchell-Reiter (1993) found that the evidence base did not identify subtle changes in patient responsiveness or color as primary early indicators of sepsis. The nurses' intuition based on experience with individual patients, however, directed them differently. The apparent contradiction between evidence (or lack thereof) and experience may stem from the difficulty defining these subtle perceptual changes. However, it is precisely the recognition of and action taken on these changes that help define clinical expertise.

The absence of difficult-to-define characteristics from the literature may reflect different assumptions underlying population and clinical medicine. The former is most often the subject of medical research. The clinical "side" of problem solving, on the other hand, is often referred to as the "art of medicine," which emphasizes experience over statistical p values. Yancy (1992, p. 365) states this best: "In good clinical practice, treatments are prescribed on the basis of various individual patient characteristics. In good clinical research, patients are assigned to treatment groups by a process explicitly designed to pay as little attention to the individual patient characteristics as medical ethics will allow." Intuition underlies decisions based on subtle, vague, or complex constellations of patient characteristics that may or may not be consciously acknowledged. Evidence-based medicine, on the other hand, is by and large derived from population-based clinical research that measures overt characteristics. In the new paradigm, students are taught to use both intuition and evidence-based medicine to solve medical problems.

SURGICAL INTUITION

Clinical intuition is the "unconscious" application of knowledge gained through experience. When used most effectively, it enhances perception and *embellishes best evidence*. Consider the following surgical script (Abernathy & Hamm, 1995, p. 100), which provides three scenarios, each increasing in complexity and the need to apply intuition to the clinical decision. In the scenarios, intuition is *combined with* evidence-based medicine to make connections between what the surgeon sees and what he or she does not see.

A 55-year-old woman with a gunshot wound in the chest presented in the emergency department. Consider what a surgeon needs to *know* to understand each of the following situations:

1. The doctor noted: she had lost 2 liters of blood, which was on her clothing, and active bleeding from the entrance wound and said, "Let's take her to the OR."
2. The doctor noted: no bleeding from the entrance wound, blood pressure of 60/palp and heart rate of 120, and said, "Let's take her to the OR."
3. The doctor noted: blood pressure okay, no bleeding from the entrance wound, but more than 100 cc out her chest tube in 20 minutes, and said, "Let's take her to the OR."

In scenario 1, even the novice medical learner can surmise that whatever is still bleeding is likely arterial and will require intervention. In scenario 2, both the more advanced learner and the expert would recognize the discordant sets of data—vitals versus physical signs. Although the patient looks stable, the patient's vitals are clues that what is "seen" is misleading. Intuition would suggest that very low blood pressure and a high pulse in a "high-risk" situation requires surgical intervention to rule out active bleeding. In scenario 3, we could infer that intuition contributed to the decision when commonly accepted guidelines were not followed. We could imagine that certain characteristics of the situation or patient—perhaps the location of the wound or the patient looking a little pale or slightly agitated—led to the decision to operate, even if these features were not recognized overtly by the surgeon. If intuition is dismissed by the surgeon in favor of the best evidence *and* the bleeding has not stopped, the decision to not go to the OR may lead to the patient's death.

RADIOLOGY AND SEARCH SUPERIORITY

Intuition or rapid metacognition is especially helpful to expert clinical problem solvers in specialty areas where incoming data may be more uniform or specific. Take, for example, the area of visual scanning, a data search task common to radiologists. As in the previous surgical example, intuition relies on pattern recognition. Some researchers posit that experts who rely on visual data can create a visual picture from stimuli before they actually see it (Resnick, 2004). For example, before expert radiologists read a CT scan or an X-ray, they have the expected picture in their heads based on experience. In these situations, they may "sense" that the stimulus (e.g., through pattern recognition) is abnormal but don't actually *see it* until they report it. The implication for medicine and medical education is clear, especially for those specialties that rely on visual data such as radiology. Novice learners must become proficient and then expert in recognizing these patterns and ultimately relying on their intuition (or mastery of visual pattern recognition) to solve clinical problems.

There is some evidence that radiologists as a group *intuit* abnormalities in the films they observe and that these intuitions lead them to identify abnormalities. They are said to have developed expertise in visual scanning or "search superiority" (Norman, Muzzin, Somers, & Rosenthal, 1992). This intuitive sense evident in expert radiologists "functions automatically to draw attention to the abnormal configurations in the radiograph gestalt" (Norman et al., 1992, p. 205; see also chapter 2).

PRIMARY CARE

Intuition is the close companion of metacognition in the experiential repertoire of the primary care physician. Its importance is enhanced by the doctor's capability to develop and maintain a relationship with the patient. Often, the power of intuition grows from reflections about the complex patterns of behaviors, perspectives, and feelings that constitute these relationships. Consider how intuition, based largely on the physician's relationship with the patient, enhances the physician's problem-solving ability and the outcomes of the following encounter.

> On my first day back from seeing patients after vacation, a 64-year-old male for whom I've provided care for 10 years came in with a chief complaint of leg weakness that had developed the day after a motor vehicle accident on July 4. He had no head injury or loss of consciousness. However, about 2 minutes into the interview, *I knew that something serious was wrong.*
>
> He described weakness in his legs, left greater than right, that was interfering with his work as a grocery stocker for a bread company. He was having difficulty squatting or lifting. He had been to urgent care on July 13, and they felt that he had "back pain" and sent him to physical therapy. He had had a physical therapy assessment that morning, so I called the physical therapist and asked about her assessment, knowing they usually do a very good job picking up weakness, and they felt that he had not been weak.
>
> However, *I was convinced even with all this information that he had a serious problem.* I did a careful physical exam and neurological exam and did document his left-leg weakness. However, his reflexes were normal, including absence of a Babinski response (primitive reflex) that would go along with a central nervous system injury.

I ordered an MRI of his head, and 2 days later he was diagnosed on MRI with a huge, chronic subdural hematoma and had surgery the next day. He's recovering at home. (UMMS Faculty Member, personal communication, September 15, 2005)

On reflection, this primary care physician was able to articulate the influence of his relationship with the patient on his intuitive decision to order the MRI. He states, "I've thought a lot about my quick and accurate assessment despite the contradictory assessments of others and my own observations that went counter to my assessment. I believe that my *long-term relationship* with this stoic, hardworking man, with particular attention to his level of concern, *was behind my intuition.*" This example of intuitive problem solving clearly demonstrates that relationship is an essential aspect of experience that must be considered along with evidence in expert primary care problem solving.

As discussed already, during problem solving, intuition relies on rapid pattern recognition. In the previous surgical example, the pattern or gestalt being "disturbed" included mostly physical and physiologic features of the patient and environment. In the primary care examples, the patterns that are "disturbed" or influential in decision making include the complexities of known and expected behaviors, personality traits, and attitudes as well as feelings of both the doctor and the patient. These patterns are developed over the period of the relationship, whether short or long. In the previous example, the physical evidence—gathered either by other health care professionals or by the doctor himself—did not warrant further investigation of the complaint. The MRI saved the patient's life and was ordered because of the doctor's intuition. The intuitive feelings were informed largely by his relationship with the patient.

Under the umbrella of relationship is perspective taking. In the previous example, the primary care physician rapidly and unconsciously took the patient's perspective in relation to the complaint. If it weren't *serious pain,* this patient wouldn't complain. Intuition often includes taking the perspective of the patient and of others "in and outside of" the exam room to make the correct diagnosis. Consider the role of perspective taking in intuition in the following case.

An 18-year-old female's mother called saying the child had suddenly lost use of both arms and was having trouble walking. The nurse who had answered the phone told me the story, and my *initial reaction* was to have her tell them to *get the girl to the ER,* thinking this was a horrible case of meningitis.

However, my instinct, perhaps based on experience, was to get a little more information. I had the nurse ask, "Does she have a fever, has she been ill, does she have a rash?" The nurse repeated aloud mom's response to each question—"no" to each. I immediately got on the phone, and after a brief conversation with mom, whom I knew very well, my *gut feeling* was that the girl wasn't severely ill, so I told them to come right in to see me.

Minutes later, the girl and her parents walked in to the office, talking to each other. She stated to me that she couldn't feel her hands and that her arms and legs felt weak. It was during this discussion that I noticed she was speaking in short sentences, almost gasping for air as we talked.

I thought, "Could she be hyperventilating? And, if so, why?"

Almost instinctively, I asked the parents to leave so I could talk with the girl alone. I had her breathe into a paper bag for a few minutes, and sure enough, the sensations in her hands were back to normal. So I asked her what was going on. Was she terribly anxious about something? She told me she had sex for the first time the night before and was considering telling her parents. (UMMS Faculty Member, personal communication, August 12, 2005)

During this clinical problem-solving experience, intuition was favored over logic at several points along the way. Logic dictated the first reaction, which was diagnosis equals meningitis: get her to the ER! However, mom's responses to questioning led him to read into her perspective and decide to "get her in here" instead. Cues from the responses to specific questions as well as the *way* mom conveyed her concern and experience of the child's symptoms led to the intuitive decision to see the patient. The visit included subtle visual cues that triggered additional associations. Once the doctor saw the girl, intuition alerted him to her "odd cadence" in speech even though he never counted her respiration. Then, intuitively (without conscious thought) and perhaps as a result of previous experience with adolescents, he asked the parents to leave the room and questioned her about her anxiety. Again, there were no recognized physical signs or symptoms of anxiety.

In primary care, patients often present cues two or three steps removed from logico-deductive diagnostic thinking. The physician often "fills in the gaps" with intuition. In this interaction, the doctor intuitively had the patient come in, noticed what could be signs of hyperventilation, and asked the parents to leave the room. Might the doctor have asked himself consciously, "Could this be hyperventilation?" Regardless of the role of metacognition, intuition was instrumental in defining the clinical outcome.

INPATIENT MEDICINE

Intuition plays an important part in the decision-making process of physicians engaged in the complex interpersonal and medical context of *inpatient* care. The following case is particularly illustrative of the complexity of patient care decisions that are made in the context of teams that include students and residents typical in inpatient settings. In those contexts, the intuition of an expert faculty member is grounded in great experience with both patients and learners.

I'm thinking about a patient with many medical problems who came to see me about 1 week after discharge from a long hospitalization involving an ICU stay. He was seen by my resident in clinic, who reviewed his discharge and assessed how he'd been feeling since then. The resident presented the case to me, and we both went in to see him.

I noticed that his eye was slightly red and weepy—a clear, teary discharge. The patient noted that the one thing that really still bothered him was his eye. As often happens, for whatever reason, this was something the resident had not learned from him, though the resident had noted a slightly red eye and had dismissed it as an issue not requiring more information.

In asking the patient about his eye, he said it had started the day before discharge from the hospital and that the team hadn't been concerned but that it was in fact painful, not just scratchy, and that his vision was slightly blurred. I asked the resident to do a fluorescence exam, and, in fact, there were dendritic lesions (herpes virus infection). We sent him that day to ophthalmology.

I talked with the resident after about how to not miss such an important diagnosis and about what *made me* want to learn more. I think there were a few issues that made me *go with my "gut"* that this was not just to be dismissed "with warm compresses":

1. I knew the patient better than the resident knew him. He'd been very sick, and to come out of that illness episode complaining about his eye would be unusual. If it didn't really bother him, I think he would have been more focused on his ICU stay.
2. I also knew he had severe postherpetic neuralgia from prior shingles and, since he had been so sick, had been relatively immunosuppressed, and this might have been a reactivation, though in a different part of his body.
3. When someone has an eye problem, there are a few key questions to ask that the resident had not, specifically about orbital pain and vision change.

But it all started with an *uneasy feeling* that there was something else going on. (UMMS Faculty Member, personal communication, October 20, 2005)

The resident and the expert faculty member both noticed the "slightly red" eye, but only the more experienced physician acted on the information. As the faculty member states, the resident decided the issue did not need to be pursued. The decision to pursue it was not a "conscious" decision as such but rather an action prompted by the *intuition* that something wasn't quite right. Her stated explanation to the resident involved several pieces of data or information that led to the decision to investigate further. Some data were "intuitive" assumptions based on experience and advanced perspective taking—he had just gone through a very painful experience and wouldn't complain about something insignificant. Some of the data that prompted the decision were grounded in her knowledge base—immunosuppression—and recollection of guidelines characterizing eye pain. By her own report, the action was initiated by the uneasy gut feeling associated with intuition.

A METACOGNITIVE APPROACH

Metacognitive capabilities enable the clinician to solve problems with conscious deliberation. One important focus of deliberation is potential error that emanates from our intuitive feelings or cognitive dispositions to respond (CDR; Croskerry, 2003). Croskerry has identified 30 CDRs that can lead to diagnostic error if left unchecked. The following is a sample from Croskerry's list: *aggregate bias*—belief that aggregate data (e.g., guidelines) do not apply to your individual patient; *anchoring*—tendency to focus on salient features too early in the diagnostic process; and *gender bias*—belief that gender is a diagnostic factor when no such evidence exists (Croskerry, 2003, p. 777). Expert problem solvers must be aware of CDRs, anticipate their influence, and reflect on their potential impact on the problem-solving process. Perhaps with training and practice, the metacognitive process of bias recognition and remediation could become intuitive.

Davidson, Deuser, and Sternberg (1994) describe four steps in problem solving that include metacognitive capabilities: (a) identifying and defining the problem, (b) mentally representing the problem, (c) planning how to proceed, and (d) evaluating what you know about your performance. These steps, which are considered separately next, should be taught to and consciously practiced by novice learners as a way to improve metacognitive capabilities.

Step 1. Defining the Problem

The expert physician first encodes the relevant features of the current case and stores these features of the problem in working memory. Next, he or she retrieves from long-term memory information that is relevant to these features. A metacognitive approach to defining the problem begins with strong and deliberate recollection of past learning that stems from evidence read or direct experience with patients. In some instances, the two sources may be contradictory. Consider the following example.

> A 58-year-old male accountant sent me an e-mail stating that he was getting dizzy periodically. This had been going on for a week, and his wife, a nurse, was pestering him to get it checked out. I called him: no chest pain, no shortness of breath, and no recent illness. His past history was clean: no

hypertension or high cholesterol, no smoking, no family history of early heart disease, and no diabetes.

I brought him into the office immediately; he thought that ridiculous. His exam was completely normal. I did an ECG, and it showed he had completed a heart attack. I couldn't believe it; neither could he. I had to argue with him to go to the ER; he drove himself. He was cathed the next day and had triple bypass 3 days later. He thinks I am a genius; I thought I was lucky.

I brought him in immediately and did the ECG because of my experience with past patients. The evidence would say that he was low risk. And 99% of the time, this would apply. But it reminds me all the time that the one in one hundred chance can happen any time. (UMMS Faculty Member, personal communication, August 12, 2005)

Defining the problem in this case was the direct result of reflection on past experience despite the contradiction with best evidence. Often clinical problems have ill-defined characteristics. These characteristics may be especially ill-defined when they are relayed secondhand—by a resident, another attending, a consultant, a significant other, or an official interpreter. "Givens" can be investigated and interpreted in different ways by different reporters. Characteristics of the "presenting problem" may or may not be precisely translated in a note or over the phone.

The primary care physician has a great deal of information and knowledge about the patient that can *help or hinder* the definition of a problem. An important task is to *try* to reflect on what knowledge is relevant and what is not. During this early step, it is important to filter out the noise inherent in reflection. As every physician will testify, there is no guarantee that filtering will work. The following is an example of an expert primary care physician's challenge in determining the more and less relevant experiential data from patients.

Two years ago, my last patient of the day was an alcoholic in his late 30s. The patient I saw just before him had MS and was in acute crisis; her breathing was in trouble. I sent her to the ER. My nurse put the alcoholic patient in the exam room while the ambulance driver took my history on the MS patient.

The alcoholic patient's story was that he was lifting a new motorcycle engine into place when he developed acute left shoulder pain 4 days ago. The doctor on call had told him to take Advil. But the pain persisted. I checked him out—his shoulder exam and his cardiac exam were 100% normal.

To be safe, I did an ECG, which was completely normal. I gave him an X-ray slip and told him not to drink and so on until we could get this worked out. The next day, his wife called to say that they still hadn't gone to get the X-ray, and now he is complaining and feels terrible. My nurse told her to get him to the ER. The patient died en route.

When I decided to not admit the patient immediately, I *reflected on* the patient's history of substance abuse and noncompliance. I did the ECG because, on some level, I guess I thought about his heart. In retrospect and on reflection, I could have *logically* sent him to the ER that day (two office patients in a row to the ER—never happened before), but I didn't *believe* this was his heart on the basis of what I knew about him and the test results. I also knew he would argue with me about going to the ER because that's the type of patient he was. (UMMS Faculty Member, personal communication, August 10, 2005)

In this case, what the physician intuitively *knew* about the patient influenced his decision making and contributed *noise* that was detrimental to the problem-solving process at this earliest stage. According to Croskerry (2003), this would likely be a good example of *posterior probability error* or the tendency to be influenced by relationship and prior experience with and knowledge of the patient. Based on previous experience (i.e., relationship) with this patient, a *logical* interpretation of the situation would be that a young, sturdy patient who was lifting a motorcycle engine can't be having a myocardial infarction—must be musculoskeletal. He doesn't need to go the ER—he won't go anyway.

Gladwell (2005) feels that in problem solving, less often is more. Sometimes this refers to beliefs and feelings that are tied to the relationship as well as facts in the case. This would apply to the novice as well as the expert. A good example of the benefit of thinking *less is more* is Goldman's algorithm for chest pain in an emergent situation. It includes only three factors to be considered along with the results of an ECG: (a) unstable angina, (b) fluid in the lungs, and (c) systolic blood pressure less than 100 (Goldman et al., 1996). Combinations of the risk factors with or without a positive ECG would be handled differently. According to Goldman's algorithm, these risk factors are much more relevant or *pertinent* than risk factors like smoking, obesity, stress, and even associated symptoms such as sweating and age *for this particular episode*. This doesn't mean that overall or in the long run a patient with these other risk factors will not be more likely to have or develop cardiac problems and have a higher mortality likelihood. However, he will be less likely to die in the next 72 hours if he does not have the three previously listed results.

The implication for metacognition is clearly related to prioritizing risk factors, not simply adding them up. Prioritizing is checking your thinking by assessing the value of unequal parts on the basis of characteristics of the current situation. In this regard, too much consideration of risk factors that are less relevant to the current episode can interfere with solving the immediate problem.

Defining the problem represents the planning phase of problem solving and begins when the expert receives the chart or recognizes the patient in the waiting room. It may be influenced by anticipation or expectation based on experience or knowledge and is often initiated prior to the patient interaction. When the expert obtains the chart or the discharge note, he or she begins to activate prior knowledge and generate conditional hypotheses. These hypotheses can be influenced by many types of bias and must be checked immediately (Croskerry, 2003). It is important that defining the problem be viewed iteratively—that it could change dramatically depending on the course of the experience or interaction. To effect the required change, the student must activate other metacognitive capabilities, such as reflection and perspective taking.

Step 2. Mental Representation

As Davidson et al. (1994, p. 209) state, "After a problem is encoded, the solver must determine what is known, what is unknown, and what is being asked in the situation." The physician goes about the process of mentally representing the problem to determine where the gaps in his thinking were. An important feature is to investigate the relations among the elements as dictated by past experience. The aim of this step is to create a "mental map" of the elements' relations and the goals of the encounter.

Mental representation is an iterative process when applied to clinical problem solving. Davidson et al. (1994, p. 215) have described three metacognitive processes associated with this step: (a) *selective encoding* is the process of seeing new stimuli that had been previously been overlooked or not evident, (b) *selective combination* is putting things together that were not formerly evident, and (c) *selective comparison* involves contrasting the current patient history with the histories of past patients. The following case description illustrates the power of selective comparison. The young patient is the younger sister of the patient who was intuitively diagnosed with appendicitis in the case described at the beginning of chapter 4.

> The younger sister came in 2 years after the previously described episode with belly pain. Like her brother before her, overall she also looked fine but was tender in the lower-right quadrant. There was no knot in my stomach about her, and my intuition said she was probably fine and could be sent home to watch for signs of appendicitis. *Thinking back* on the experience I had with her brother and how mild his presentation was for appendicitis, however, I decided to send her to the ER for an ultrasound. The result was negative, she was fine—no appendicitis—and went home. (UMMS Faculty Member, personal communication, August 21, 2005)

Step 3. Planning How to Proceed

Davidson et al. (1994, p. 215) make the following observations about planning:

1. Individuals are more likely to plan in novel or complex situations.
2. Planning tends to be abstract rather than concrete.

3. Plans are revised based on how it is going.
4. Plans take time but in the long run improve efficiency.

The following clinical case illustrates the changing nature and relent-lessness often required by clinical experts in planning and managing patient care. It is particularly illustrative of multiple contextual features that must be considered in medical problem solving.

I took over a ward service last year, busy as usual, with the usual number of patients "ready for discharge and just waiting for the new attending" to come on. One was an elderly man, early 80s, admitted with syncopal episodes. Seemed he'd had a big work-up, and it looked like it might be neurogenic. He'd been started on medications, and his symptoms had improved but not completely gone away. The team was ready to discharge him the day I arrived.

When I met the patient, it was hard to get a handle on his story because he had moderate dementia. He seemed somewhat frail. I told the team I thought he could go home but wanted to review a few studies during the morning. There were some questions I had that they couldn't answer, like why he was wearing oxygen. When I went over the history I discovered that he had a positive d-dimer, ordered by a night float about 4 days earlier. I delved a little deeper and found his ECG had changed over time. I started to get worried that there might be a more serious cause.

I wanted to discharge him, the team was large, and he'd been sitting in the hospital for a few days without much happening as his medication was being adjusted. But he just wasn't getting better, and there were *unanswered questions*. I *consciously* thought about the various causes of syncope and went *systematically* through his chart trying to use the data there to rule in or out each cause. I kept coming to the *unanswered questions*—he was mildly hypoxic, his ECG had changed though he hadn't had a myocardial infarction, his d-dimer had been mildly elevated, and he wasn't better. Of course, he might never get better—he was elderly, somewhat demented, and on many medications; this might be his new baseline, but there were physiologic abnormalities that were *unexplained*.

I looked further; he'd had surgery 6 weeks ago and seemed to have been appropriately anticoagulated in the hospital and at the skilled nursing facility. Surgery could account for his elevated d-dimer, but so could a deep-vein thrombosis or pulmonary embolism (PE), which could also account for his hypoxia, ECG change, and syncope. I told the team I wanted an echo to look at his heart function. I didn't want to expose him to a dye load if I could avoid it. *They were very resistant.* I reviewed that there were real unanswered physiologic abnormalities we had to address and also that, *if we missed this, he could die,* and at the very least if he kept syncopizing at home, he'd be right back in the hospital if we hadn't addressed all potential serious issues. They finally agreed, though of course since I'm the attending, they would have had to do it anyway. He had near right-heart failure. The subsequent CT showed massive PEs and a saddle embolus. He was taken to the OR in the middle of the night. (UMMS Faculty Member, personal communication, October 20, 2005)

Problem solving often occurs in the context of a team that involves multiple providers representing many levels of experience. In this context, the planning process is interwoven with the coordination of patient care. It is ever changing and requires great attention and effective communication. In these contexts, expert planning and subsequent implementation typically involve teamwork, information gathering, reflecting, and directing others' behaviors.

Step 4. Evaluation

Once a solution is identified, checking it against other possibilities is often the key metacognitive ingredient of a successful outcome. Reviewing the thought process and ultimately the decision for evidence of accuracy and bias reflects the final step in thinking about one's thinking. Self-evaluation, including self-questioning, should occur throughout the problem-solving process (King, 1991).

The following excerpt came from an expert clinician's evaluation of a student who was identified as a *weak finisher*. Although the student demonstrated good anticipation and planning, he had great difficulty monitoring his thinking and checking or evaluating his own performance at the end of an interaction. He often experienced difficulty with premature closure:

> You need to make sure that at the end of your interview you are comfortable with the picture of the patient that you have painted. That would include (but not be limited to):
>
> - After you feel that you are finished, ask:
>   - Does this make sense?
>   - Does it make sense that this patient is dehydrated after not eating for 6 hours but with only one episode of vomiting?
>   - Does it make sense that a patient with a strep throat should be sick this long?
>   - Are these labs what I expected?
>   - Am I comfortable with this diagnosis or with this patient? Am I worried?
>   - Did I "reach" this patient? If the patient is uncomfortable or is not "buying" your diagnosis, at least rethink things.

The following exercises would be good practice. Try constructing circumstantial questions for the following symptoms to use as a check on your thinking:

- Patient has a sleep problem.
- Patient has temper tantrums. Here is a hint: Think of the ABCs (Antecedent, Behavior, Consequence).
- A patient with vomiting and diarrhea for a week (what do you want to know?).
- Make up your own chief complaint and figure out what you need to know.

Reflection is a good tool to help you know when you need to expand your differential or rethink the case. It's a good tool to prevent premature closure.

SUMMARY

Intuition and metacognition are critical ingredients of clinical problem solving. Intuition relies on unconscious pattern recognition related to many modes of experiencing the environment, including visual-perceptual and social-relational. The latter may include the ability to take the patient's (or family member's) perspective. Metacognition centers around the abilities to reflect on the nature of the problem and biases, mentally represent the problem, plan, and self-evaluate. Both intuition and metacognition shape the recognition, selection, and interpretation of *best evidence* available to the physician. The capabilities that constitute each are separated by time and level of consciousness (see Figure 1.1 in chapter 1). The expert clinician uses and requires both sets of capabilities. The new paradigm in medical education focuses on the development of these capabilities through lifelong learning.

CHAPTER SEVEN

Communication and the Physician–Patient Relationship

INTRODUCTION

In chapter 6, metacognition and intuition were discussed in relation to clinical problem solving related to patient care. In this chapter, another competency defined by the Accreditation Council of Graduate Medical Education—interpersonal communication—is analyzed in relation to its metacognitive and intuitive elements. Patients' perspectives are critical elements of strategic knowledge (see chapter 3 on metacognitive capabilities) that should be elicited to enhance interpersonal communication. Metacognitive techniques such as self-questioning by the student or physician can be combined with direct questioning of the patient to better understand differences in perspective that influence communication in the doctor–patient relationship. The idea that emotional intelligence, as defined in the literature, *is* emotional metacognition is raised in this chapter. The act of apology is used as an example of emotional intelligence that requires metacognitive capabilities. The importance of first impressions (a phenomenon that grows out of intuition) and their relationship to outcomes of communication, such as patient satisfaction and stereotyping, are discussed.

METACOGNITION AND COMMUNICATION

"I can't believe it could be cancer." The 37-year-old mother of three had scheduled the appointment with her primary care physician to discuss tubal ligation as a birth control method and receive results of screening tests. To her dismay, results of the mammogram identified the presence a suspicious lump. Dr. Jones, an experienced obstetrician, has the challenging task of informing this patient of the test results. He responds to her emotional expression of disbelief with a calm demeanor: "We will do everything we can to help you through this." He pauses and waits for her reply. She sighs and fidgets with a tissue she is holding. In a few moments that would seem an eternity to a novice interviewer, she follows with, "I should have found it earlier." Dr. Jones says, "You did all the right things—regular breast self-exams and screening mammograms. It's not your fault that it is there now. We have found it early, and that is very good." They both pause. Dr. Jones *sees* that she is thinking it is cancer. "This is most likely noncancerous. We don't know for sure, so we need to take a closer look." During the next 3 minutes, the doctor elicits more of the patient's concerns and addresses them. At times he looks at the situation from the patient's point of view. At other times, he checks his own behavior to make sure he is not overinforming, making assumptions about her feelings and thoughts, or saying the wrong things.

On the contrary, novices—students who are not intuitive communicators or metacognitively capable—*appear* to be egocentric and uncaring with their patients. During clinical clerkships, their preceptors who observe them with patients may feel that they "talk too much." One preceptor described John, a third-year student who could not monitor or regulate his communication, as emitting "background noise that he can't turn off." The same preceptor said that John "did too much out-loud thinking, almost rambling to the patient about what was going on in his head." This nonreflective, egocentric approach to communication detracts from achieving goals related to the three functions of the medical interview (Lazare, Putnam, & Lipkin, 1995). Straying away from the patient and his or her needs most often leads to (a) incomplete and inaccurate data gathering, (b) overinforming while trying to educate the patient, and (c) the patient feeling "not listened to" and a victim of an uncaring attitude.

John must learn, as Dr. Jones has, to elicit and convey an understanding of the patient's perspective. He must use this understanding to monitor the information he provides and to recognize and address the patient's concerns. Like other novice learners and some more experienced physicians, John has a tendency to preempt the patient's offering of the "chief concern" with information on "how it must feel" and then promptly informs (rather than empathizes) as a method of allaying the concern.

In the previous example, Dr. Jones recognized verbal and nonverbal cues that signaled the patient's emotional distress. It is a common pitfall for many novice and even experienced interviewers to neglect these cues. Consciously or unconsciously, it is perceived as far "safer" and more efficient to attribute feelings and inform than to elicit feelings and empathize. Novice students who do not possess metacognitive capabilities unconsciously "miss" or consciously "ignore" important verbal and nonverbal cues that indicate a patient's emotional response. They experience particular difficulty when the patient has a strong emotional reaction to something that is said or done. Their teachers and colleagues typically describe them as having "a very difficult time connecting with the patient."

The practice of medicine requires making decisions and taking action on the basis of an accurate account of the presenting problem and its impact on the patient's life. With respect to communication, this is completed by gathering information (i.e., history), developing the relationship, and educating the patient (Lazare et al., 1995). This can be completed only by gaining a deep understanding of the patient's concerns (i.e., feelings about the problem) and beliefs (e.g., reasons for and outcomes related to the problem). In addition, the physician must assess the credibility (reliability and validity) of the patient's story. The physician's effectiveness in accomplishing these goals is dependent on knowledge of his or her communication style and ability to regulate his or her own (and monitor the patient's) communication behavior during the interaction. Obtaining a deep understanding of self and other and monitoring an interaction through reflection and perspective taking is metacognition applied to communication. Metacognition plays a critical role in diagnosis, treatment, and prevention of disease and underpins the physician–patient relationship.

The unintended result of John's inability to view the patients' perspectives is confusion, inattention, and feelings of powerlessness on the part of the patient. The dissatisfied patient will label the student doctor as not listening and uncaring.

During clinical learning experiences, novice learners will benefit from asking themselves the following questions to guide metacommunication before, during, and after an interview:

- Am I providing information that this patient needs (how do I know)?
- What does this patient think is happening to him or her and why (reasons for illness or potential outcomes)?
- What are his or her concerns (deepest fears)?
- How accurate is this patient's story (what is my evidence)?
- How do I feel about the patient and his or her condition (do I have a bias)?
- How confident am I that I can help him or her (what do I know or need to know)?

- What does this patient know about this condition (how is his or her knowledge different than mine)?

John participated in a series of tutorials to improve his metacognitive capabilities during the clinical years. He watched himself and the patient on videotape after encounters with standardized patients. He would be asked what he was thinking and what he thought the patient was thinking and feeling. The patient would then tell him what he or she was thinking and feeling. These sessions were used to improve reflection, self-assessment, and perspective-taking capabilities. In one of these guided reflection sessions, he characterized his patient encounter as a "blind race" and stated that he "almost appears to be strong-arming the patient." He initially set two goals: (a) allow the patient to finish what he or she is saying and (b) allow the patient to dictate his or her own agenda. Recognizing his inability to take the patient's perspective was an essential first step to changing John's behavior.

One important goal in perspective taking that influences the physician's ability to educate is estimating the patient's level of knowledge. This can be heavily influenced by the physician's own knowledge. Nickerson, Baddeley, and Freeman (1987, p. 257) state, "We use our own knowledge as the basis for a default model of what other people know. . . . We then use any awareness that our own knowledge is unusual in specific ways to modify our model of what the typical other person knows." Many studies have demonstrated this problem of "false consensus" (Ross, Greene, & House, 1977).

False consensus can have a major impact in medicine. The default model—what the physician knows—can be very different from what a typical patient knows. It often interferes with the accurate understanding of the patient's story. An indicator of the magnitude of this discrepancy in understanding is the oft-reported finding that patients are dissatisfied with the physician's use of medical jargon (Duffy, Gordon, Whelan, Cole-Kelly, & Frankel, 2004). Many providers would do a better job of perspective taking and educating if they monitored their use of language and periodically checked the patient's understanding of what was being said. Students can develop these metacognitive skills in their early interactions with patients.

PERSPECTIVE TAKING AS THE FOUNDATION OF "METACOMMUNICATION"

Perspective is an individual's viewpoint in general or that of a particular situation, event, or person. As such, it involves a metacognitive assessment and evaluation (determination of importance). The ability to take (actually attempt to approximate) another person's perspective develops over time. Developmental psychologists have demonstrated that this ability evolves from egocentricism at the earliest stage in childhood (dedifferentiation of self from others) through recognition of independence of others yet believing that "my way is the best way" in adolescence to the ability to respectfully view the world from the eyes of others (Selman, 1971). The metacognitive ability of perspective taking underlies many critical communication skills, such as negotiating, empathizing, and educating. It also underlies other critical aspects of expertise, such as professionalism.

AN EXAMPLE OF POOR PERSPECTIVE TAKING IN THE CLINICAL ENCOUNTER

The following transcript of an interaction between a student and a standardized patient illustrates how novice students can lose sight of the patient's perspective and agenda as they make an effort to inform and educate the patient. In the interaction, the student fails to recognize verbal and nonverbal cues exhibited by the patient that should warn the interviewer of this *miscommunication*. The student does to the patient what he may have experienced himself in the curriculum—he overinforms:

STUDENT: Good morning, Ms. Starr. I see from your chart that you're here for a possible pregnancy. I understand you did a home pregnancy test that was positive and the urine that you dropped off was also positive for pregnancy.

PATIENT: (Sigh . . . looking at the floor) I was hoping it wouldn't be—so I wouldn't have to deal with this. I just don't know what to do.

STUDENT: Well, let me tell you your options. Number one, you can have the baby. And I see from your chart that you are healthy. You're on no medications. You don't have any allergies. And you have no significant past medical history. So we could assume that you would have a very healthy baby. Another option would be to put the child up for adoption. And the third option would be to terminate the pregnancy. And the issue there would be to find out how far along you are. When was your last menstrual period?

PATIENT: Ah . . . (hesitant) it was 6 weeks ago.

STUDENT: It was 6 weeks ago, so you do have a little time to decide.

PATIENT: The thing is, I still wouldn't know what to do. My boyfriend is going to go along with whatever I decide.

STUDENT: Well, okay. Let me tell you a little more about your options. If you do decide to have the baby, there is an ob/gyn doctor whom I could refer you to right here in this building. And if you decided to do that you would have to start taking folic acid—5 to 10 milligrams per day. You would have to start doing that now. And I don't know much about arranging for adoption myself, but I could refer you to Planned Parenthood. And if not Planned Parenthood, maybe one of those anti–planned parenthood organizations could help you also. And if you choose to terminate, we would probably have to do a D & C. We don't have any RU-486 in the office, and it's too late to use high-dose estrogen. And again I could refer you to Planned Parenthood for a possible termination. I've been down there, and it's a really nice clinic, so I think they'd take good care of you.

PATIENT: Oh . . . ah . . . this is all too overwhelming for me. I don't know. I just don't know . . . (sigh).

STUDENT: Well, I think you should discuss it with your boyfriend. I realize it's a lot to take in. If we could meet back up in a week and discuss what your decision is, and meanwhile I'd like to give you some information on Planned Parenthood. And I think it would be a good idea to give them a call this week.

PATIENT: Okay.

STUDENT: Okay. Thanks.

EMOTIONAL INTELLIGENCE

Emotional intelligence *is* emotional metacognition. It represents a strategic approach to managing one's own and the other's emotions (Matthews, Zeidner, & Roberts, 2002). It includes both executive and regulatory functions and, often early in the process, relies on intuition. A metacognitive approach to emotions can enhance communication and the doctor–patient relationship. Social awareness and relationship management are the key features of emotional intelligence as defined by Goleman (1995). An early proponent of emotional intelligence, Bar-On has identified interpersonal capabilities, such as empathy and social responsibility, as important subcomponents (Bar-On, 2000). Negotiation is another communication skill that requires metacognition. It involves recognizing and reinforcing the patient's perspective in relation to your own, educating, and compromising when necessary.

THE EXAMPLE OF APOLOGY

Taking another's perspective, or recognizing and understanding the impact of verbal and nonverbal behavior on that person, is a prerequisite to higher-order communication. Empathy and negotiation have been cited as examples. Another example of communication that requires meta-cognition is apology. Apology can be defined as "an encounter between two parties in which one party, the offender, acknowledges responsibility for an offense or grievance and expresses regret or remorse to a second party, the aggrieved" (Lazare, 2004). Acknowledging responsibility for a behavior that is "perceived" by the patient to be offensive first requires that the physician "stand in that patient's shoes," a truly metacognitive operation. Second, it requires that the physician accept rather than reject the validity of the patient's perspective. Finally, it involves valuing the dignity of the patient and/or the relationship with him or her. Consider the following scenario in which the preceptor modeled appropriate apology for the student.

> *This middle-aged executive was referred to the office for back pain and is sitting in the exam room sternly staring out the window as the doctor and the student enter.*

DOCTOR: Hello Ms. Hunt. You were referred to us by Dr. Jones for . . .

PATIENT: Do you know how long I've been waiting? Over 2 hours. You're not the only one who's busy, you know. I'm busy too. I can't afford to just sit around here waiting to see someone. I came in here sick and now I even feel sicker!

DOCTOR: I'm very sorry that we made you wait so long. That is certainly not acceptable. I will address this problem with the appropriate people as soon as we are done. I will understand if you have to leave right now, and we could schedule another appointment as soon as possible. Or I could make a phone call to let someone know why you are late if that would help.

The response involves important steps that the preceptor can model for and later reflect on, with the student. These steps are (a) identifying and controlling your initial affective response to the patient's angry words, (b) taking her perspective, and (c) formulating a plan to address her anger, offer restitution, and move the interaction to the health-related agenda.

Recognizing that one's tendency is to get angry or to self-justify in response to anger is the first step in the metacognitive process. Controlling that tendency and instead trying to achieve some common ground with the patient will require the second step: to take the patient's perspective. Regardless of the appropriateness of the patient's response, she does have "a right to be angry." Next, the plan to address her anger would most likely include apology—accepting responsibility for the "offensive" action of being part of a system that causes her to wait an extraordinary amount of time. The patient expects some form of reparation, so the apology should offer "payback options" as well.

A WORD ABOUT TEAMWORK

Communicating effectively with team members is an area that demands great metacognitive capability. Scardamalia has coined the term "collective cognitive responsibility" to represent the ideal functioning of expert teams. She describes this as "collective responsibility for understanding what is happening, for staying cognitively on top of events as they unfold" (Scardamalia, 2002, p. 2). This represents the application of metacognition to physician–team member interactions. It is the application of shared perspective taking, reflection, and other important metacognitive skills. It also can represent the application of shared problem solving if that is the task of the team.

INTUITION AND THE DOCTOR–PATIENT RELATIONSHIP

The ease and "consciousness" with which perspective taking occurs will determine whether the capability to take the patient's perspective is largely intuitive or metacognitive. The act of communication between human beings is an important component of learning about how to interact with others in the future (Lave & Wenger, 1990). According to some researchers, reading patient cues demands a conscious awareness of what the other is doing during the course of interaction. Other researchers, however, conclude that much of the interaction takes place at the unconscious or intuitive level. For example, Resnick concludes that people *sense* visual characteristics or changes without actually seeing them (Resnick, 2004). In his study, subjects were shown alternating similar pictures with minor differences, and many responded that they "sensed they were different" without actually visually experiencing or expressing the differences. In a similar way, Abernathy and Hamm state that an intuitive surgeon can "see into the belly. . . . Without laboratory or x-ray data, and simply with a brief history and a careful abdominal exam, they know what is happening with astounding accuracy" (Abernathy & Hamm, 1995, p. 3).

Simons believes that this *sensing* is really a form of seeing without verification (in Winerman, 2005). Whereas intuition involves spontaneous and often unconscious recognition of physical symptoms as well as a patient's interpersonal characteristics and features, metacognition serves to verify their presence and check their validity. This leads to further learning.

CONCEPT OF "THIN SLICES"

Intuition gained through the doctor–patient relationship is often essential to medical expertise. A growing literature is demonstrating the persuasive power, validity, and lasting effects of "first impressions." Instinctively, we "size up" someone we meet and determine if he or she is a danger and perhaps even how much we will "like" him or her. In the first few seconds, we even estimate personality characteristics, such as responsibility and trustworthiness. For example, Ambady and Rosenthal found that high school and college students evaluated teachers in the first 30 seconds (or less) of exposure (nonverbal) the same as they did at the end of a course (Ambady & Rosenthal, 1993). They refer to this as "thin slicing." In a follow-up study, Ambady and Gray (2002) correlated "thin-sliced" evaluation with what students learned from the teacher and found a positive relationship.

The implications of thin slicing for establishing a doctor–patient relationship and for patient education are far reaching. From a medical education point of view, we must ask, Can thin-sliced evaluation of people be modified and enhanced, or is it based on "fixed" personality traits? If it can be modified, will the doctor–patient relationship, patient education, and disease prevention be positively influenced? How one prepares for or anticipates first impressions may be important to this discussion.

There is little doubt that *intuition* or *rapid metacognition* can have a very powerful influence on our impressions of people. Ambady and Rosenthal's convincing studies lead to conclusions that people tend to form fairly accurate and valid perceptions of others based on only seconds of observation or interaction (Ambady & Rosenthal, 1992, 1993). Researchers have demonstrated that these first impressions are based on a host of verbal and nonverbal cues that are emitted by those being observed (Baron & Boudreau, 1987). During *everyday interactions* with others, we cultivate and trust our ability to form first impressions and make snap judgments. It is probably a survival mechanism that has its roots in instinctual behavior. When one is faced by another who is about to inflict harm, intuition becomes an escape mechanism.

The evidence of our ability to intuitively read someone—including the observance of nonverbal cues—has convinced some researchers that this intuitive ability renders conscious awareness of nonverbal behavior unnecessary and perhaps even invalidating. In this regard, Ambady and Gray state, "Taken together, these results indicate that a careful, deliberative strategy of interpreting nonverbal cues is not only unnecessary but may actually be somewhat of a hindrance to accurate judgment" (Ambady & Gray, 2002, p. 950). Thier findings on the validity of intuition should press physicians to recognize and give serious consideration to intuitive feelings about the patient (e.g., patient's likelihood to follow through with a treatment regimen).

The concepts of thin slicing and awareness can be brought into conscious deliberation through metacognition. In some situations this can lead to more valid perceptions. In an interesting illustration of this, Gottman instructed people to go into dorm rooms to form opinions of students' personalities based on their perceptions of the surroundings. In a real sense, they were asked to "think about their thinking"—to question their assumptions (in Gladwell, 2005). The exposure with instructions to be aware increased the validity of perceptions about others.

Not only should physicians in training recognize when they are forming first impressions of patients, but they must also realize that each new patient is thin slicing his or her own behavior and that the relationship as perceived from both sides will be based on these first impressions. These impressions will include both verbal and nonverbal physician behavior and can significantly impact medical outcomes and the doctor–patient relationship. The clues as to what patients thin slice may be found in studies of doctor–patient communication and patient satisfaction. For example, Levinson, Roter, Mullooly, Dull, and Frankel (1997) found that surgeons who were sued less often offered more "orienting" comments (e.g., "I'll leave time for your questions"), offered verbal prompts (e.g., "Go on, tell me about . . . "), were funny, and allowed the interaction to go on longer. The differences between the two groups of surgeons consist of the communication process and not the content of what is said.

To further illustrate the importance of process over content in the formation of first impressions, Ambady et al. "content filtered" (garbled) the same videotaped interactions analyzed by Levinson et al. (1997) and had patients rate the physicians on characteristics such as warmth and anxiousness using tone only (Ambady et al., 2002). They found that the two groups of surgeons could be differentiated (more sued vs. less sued) on these characteristics regardless of *what* they were saying. The *higher-sued* group tended to be rated as more dominant and less concerned about the patient's problem. Thus, tone may be a signal for warmth and trust; gestures and facial features may signify extraversion, which is positively evaluated by patients as a sign of caring attitude. These traits may be most salient to the intuitive self. They may also be behaviors that could be modified through metacognition and medical education.

Intuition alone may not be the most effective way to make decisions about patients and their care. Studies and common sense tell us that intuitive impressions that underlie decisions don't always pan out.

This is evident in many arenas where we are expected to form judgments about people. As Glovich states with reference to the medical school applicant interview, "No unstructured interview for any kind of position—graduate school, medical school, the military or professional jobs—has anything but low validity for predicting the interviewee's future performance" (in Greer, 2005, p. 59). Anticipating and checking intuitive impressions about medical school applicants, patients, and others with whom we interact is likely to help us achieve greater success in our interpersonal endeavors.

Some would argue that interpersonal intuition derives from a desire to understand or make sense of a chaotic world of interpersonal and cultural differences. It may actually represent an unconscious need to establish patterns or prescriptions for interpersonal behavior based on experience. It is an adaptation to a world where relationships with others are so complex (or in some cases random) that trying to figure all of them out would paralyze the decision-making process as it relates to others. A premium is placed on efficiency and expedience. Intuitive responses to others are integral to decision making in medicine, where time is a commodity, survival of the patient is at stake, and emotions on all sides are running high. Often it is an adaptive response and linked to positive outcomes.

Although adaptive in many instances, interpersonal intuition can also be maladaptive. As Glovich states, "Intuition leads us astray because it's not very good at picking up flaws in the evidence" (in Greer, 2005, p. 60). It tends to operate in the global domain—effective in recognizing and synthesizing general similarities but ineffective in recognizing and differentiating on the basis of nuances. This tendency toward generalization synthesis will lead to medical errors in problem solving. It will also result in stereotyping patients and failure to establish appropriate relationships. As Glovich states, "The intuitive system will be faulty when the world conspires against us to present information that is misleading" (in Greer, 2005, p. 59). In the world of medicine, such misleading information is common and can negatively influence the outcomes of patient care.

SUMMARY

The expert knows when to rely on intuition and when to use metacognitive abilities to elicit diagnostic data, educate the patient, and foster the doctor–patient relationship. Intuition, in particular, underlies valuable first impressions, and thin slicing can often facilitate the development of relationships. However, relying on intuition alone can create a heuristic or worldview that is easily swayed by bias and not very efficient in the long run. It is present oriented and easily misled by emotions. Because interpersonal interactions and relationships in medicine are often characterized by intense emotions related to pain, unreal expectations for health, addiction, or loss, they may be highly susceptible to the negative influences of intuition on the physician's perception, such as bias and stereotyping. Metacognitive capabilities such as perspective taking and reflection can serve as checks on interpersonal intuition by *weeding out* stereotype and controlling bias.

CHAPTER EIGHT

Professionalism

INTRODUCTION

In this chapter, metacognition is described as a critical capability in the development of professionalism. In chapters 6 and 7, the Accreditation Council of Graduate Medical Education's (ACGME's) competency areas of patient care and interpersonal communication were discussed in relation to metacognition. Once again, in this chapter the value of metacognition in the achievement of a key ACGME competency area is discussed. This chapter describes the renewed interest in professionalism as an outcome of medical education. The case is made for focusing the teaching of professionalism on the underlying thought processes (identity, perspective taking, reflection, and self-regulation) rather than specific behaviors (e.g., wearing a white coat and answering a page). Checking intuition for stereotyping is proposed. Guidance is offered for developing students' metacognitive capabilities related to several key professional attributes, including respect, honesty and integrity, and altruism.

> We, as the first physicians of the twenty-first century, will strive to hold ourselves to the highest standards. . . . We will treat our patients with empathy and respect and will work to establish open relationships characterized by honesty and trust. . . . We pledge to hold ourselves to the highest standards in our professional and personal lives . . . while maintaining an awareness of our strengths and limitations.
>
> *Declaration of Aspirations: The Oath of the University of Massachusetts Medical School (UMMS) Class of 2000*

PROFESSIONALISM REVISITED

During the first decade of the 21st century, professionalism has received a lot of attention as a required competency in medicine. In the broadest sense, professionalism entails honesty, caring, and responsibility in the relationship between doctor and patient. This includes a commitment to gaining and maintaining medical competence and applying this competence in an ethical and proactive way to benefit the patient.

The relative lack of attention to professionalism as a core competency in medicine during the latter part of the 20th century may be attributed to a diminution of the term. Wear and Castellani lament that the term "professional development" had become so amorphous as to refer to "CME, faculty development, career planning or even seminars in CV construction or how to get published" (Wear & Castellani, 2000, p. 602). The ethical, fraternal, other-centered, and self-regulatory aspects of professionalism aspired to in the UMMS students oath had been obscured and minimized by the mechanical, "job training" aspects of being a medical professional.

By the time the UMMS class of 2000 had entered medical school, efforts were already under way at many major medical schools and organizations to restore the integrity and enhance the teaching of medical professionalism. In the 1990s, the American Board of Internal Medicine initiated Project Professionalism (1995). With a focus on the doctor–patient relationship, they defined the following characteristics of professional behavior: altruism, accountability, excellence, duty, honor and integrity, and respect for others. Around the same time, the ACGME defined "professionalism outcomes" for residency training. They included specific competencies in the following areas: respect, compassion, integrity, subordination of self-interest to the needs of patients and society, commitment to excellence and lifelong learning, commitment to ethical principles related to patient care and the business of medicine, and sensitivity to differences, including patient's culture, age, gender, and disabilities (ACGME, 2005).

At the turn of the 21st century, medical schools began to adopt recommendations from the project and to build a curricular focus for the concept. In 2000, a special issue of *Academic Medicine* was devoted to professionalism and medical education (Calleigh, 2000). In that issue, major articles appeared, describing professionalism and calling for curriculum reform in this area. The reform efforts that have expanded across the medical education continuum focus on defining and evaluating behaviors associated with professionalism. Simply focusing on the behaviors, however, does not adequately ensure the depth of understanding necessary to deal with new professional challenges for generations of physicians to come. The focus on professionalism as a competency in medical education must consider the underlying metacognitive processes. Once these processes have been defined, novel approaches to teaching and curriculum reform that transcend the content of professionalism can be implemented.

PROFESSIONAL IDENTITY

From a metacognitive standpoint, professionalism implies collective identity and a commitment to regulation of values and behaviors at the self and group levels. In essence, professional identity is *collective metacognition* and significantly influences professional behavior. For many, it is the source of shared values that guides individual behaviors and serves as an inspiration for using those behaviors. Identity with a professional group may also provide feelings of intrinsic satisfaction and belongingness as well as commitment and responsibility (Starr, Ferguson, Haley, & Quirk, 2003). Possessing the metacognitive capabilities to reflect on the personal nature of one's group identity contributes significantly to the establishment of a professional identity.

Once identity is established (or renewed), it is the concept of oath or self-regulation in medicine that binds participants together and engenders the public's trust. "Without the Oath," says Pellegrino, "the doctor is a skilled technician or laborer whose knowledge fits him for an occupation but not a profession" (Pellegrino, 2002, p. 379). In essence, the oath defines the collective and fraternal nature of professionalism among physicians. The desire (or value) and the capability to uphold the standards of the group (i.e., components of self-regulation) are essential to the practice of professionalism.

Establishing and maintaining a professional identity, then, requires the capabilities to reflect on, assess, and modify one's values, attitudes, and behavior in relation to those of the profession. This requires "collective perspective taking" and motivation to belong to the group. Unprofessional behavior by medical students often begins with failure to establish collective identity with the medical profession. The following case of unprofessional behavior represents an unusual and extreme example.

Joan was a clinical student who was labeled initially as "an attitude problem" that escalated to a characterization as "unprofessional" by clerkship faculty and directors. On the one hand, many rated her communication with patients very highly. She was generally commended for her ability to establish relationships with her patients. One preceptor noted that she "spent a lot of time with her patients and gave useful feedback to the treatment team." He also said that "she was eager to learn and interested in her patients, established rapport with her patients, and was thorough and complete in her write-ups." Because she was bilingual in Spanish and English, she was also described as "culturally proficient." Another preceptor stated that "she is a remarkable person who will do well in medicine as her database grows and her clinical reasoning matures." During the 4-week clinical skills rotation, she exhibited superb communication skills with her patients. She mastered advanced skills such as delivering bad news and interviewing elderly patients with multiple complaints. Her line of questioning, verbal following techniques, and transitions were superb.

Several faculty however, noted problems with her initiative and her interactions with peers and faculty. This represented the "darker side" of her professional identity. A clerkship director observed that she was late to the clerkship orientation and to several workshops in the core curriculum. Two attendings in another clerkship stated that "she was hesitant in the group and seemed to hold back." Another noted "that she may be shy and that she was somewhat difficult to engage in discussion." One clerkship director was particularly disturbed by some of her behaviors that were thought to be unprofessional. In the clerkship, she often exhibited unusual, quizzical expressions in response to faculty questions and "exuded flat affect." When provided with this feedback based on observations, she responded, "This is who I am." When asked why "it is who you are only with faculty and not patients," she stated matter-of-factly, "That's the way I've been taught to act with patients."

She demonstrated an uncaring attitude toward her teachers and toward medicine. She expressed no problem with how others *in the profession* were seeing her because she explicitly stated that she did not share their values. She often became very closed, saying very little, breaking eye contact, and giving one-word responses to questions. "She seems angry," was a comment made by more than one faculty member. In perhaps the most telling of comments that reflected a lack of collective identity with the medical profession and her role, she stated that "my interactions with patients are an act." She also stated, "I do not like working with patients—it's my job." By her own admission, Joan did not consciously possess the metacognitive skills needed to be professional: "I can't reflect, I am not a good communicator, I don't identify my feelings, I can't assess myself."

Joan was perceived as unprofessional because she failed to identify with the profession—to share and be motivated by its values. She did not have the shared goals to compare with her reflections or the criteria to judge her self-assessments. A key feature of her lack of identity was her lack of intrinsic goal directedness. She stated, "I don't have goals. I don't think that way." A thorough neuropsychological exam of Joan revealed no underlying pathology. The evaluator referred to her as pleasant and cooperative with normal affect and very mild attention and information-processing difficulties.

Joan viewed taking care of patients as a "job" and failed to see medicine as her chosen profession. She could "act the part" with patients but could not express true altruism or empathy. She stated that she could not reflect or self-assess and had no goals with which to compare to those of the medical profession. She was motivated to become a member by extrinsic rewards (i.e., meeting the requirements of clerkships, medical school, and then residency) yet felt no identification with the profession. She felt no bond with faculty who represented the profession and admitted she had no interest in the profession other than as a job.

Joan was an outlier whose lack of identification with the profession, its values, and its culture constituted unprofessional behavior. A greater number of students, residents, and practicing physicians do express identification with the values and goals of the profession but cannot apply metacognitive capabilities necessary to regulate their professional behaviors.

COLLECTIVE PERSPECTIVE TAKING AND REGULATION

From a social metacognitive perspective, regulation should be applied by the individual to the professional group to which he or she belongs. Determining the validity and reliability of one's own knowledge and the knowledge base of one's profession are integral parts of lifelong learning. The capability to critically assess and scrutinize the knowledge base that lies at the very foundation of the profession to which one belongs is integral to professionalism. This is referred to as sociologic consciousness or "the ability to *see through* social structures, taken for granted knowledge and methods, and institutional practices so that none of these moves to a level beyond critical scrutiny" (Wear & Castellani, 2000, p. 608). Wear and Castellani (2000, p. 603) declare that students must learn to "think critically about themselves and their profession" as well as to recognize limits of both. With respect to the latter, they refer to the " deepest assumptions" underlying a profession as the assumptions about the knowledge base of the profession (p. 604). The implication for medicine as well as other professions is that the knowledge base is fallible and ever changing.

Regulation also should apply to self in relation to the medical profession. An essential capability of professionalism is acceptance of one's role and regulation of role-related behaviors within the group. Consider the following account of a resident who could not regulate her professional role-related behaviors as documented by the resident education director at the health center.

> This highly motivated and bright resident is bilingual and has medical skill well beyond her level of training. However, she takes on more responsibility than is appropriate. Initially, she ordered an epidural on an obstetrical patient without consulting her attending first. When the attending found out, she informed the resident that she, the attending, needed to be in the

hospital for this procedure and would come in immediately. The attending clearly instructed the resident to wait until she arrived. She could formulate a management plan but needed to wait for the attending before initiating. When the attending arrived 20 minutes later, the epidural had been performed. The patient's condition had not changed. The resident had asked one of the attending's colleagues to cover. (UMMS Faculty Member, personal communication, December 17, 2003)

The resident clearly understood the rules that were made explicit by the supervising attending over the telephone. However, she decided to supersede the directive from her supervisor and institute her own policy. In this instance, she failed not only to see her supervisor's perspective but also to see the perspective of the professional group to which she belonged—its values and beliefs about the attending–resident relationship. Professional identity involves understanding the concept of responsibility and how it relates to role and following instructions from superiors. Not reflecting on how one behaves in relation to the rules and standards of the group results in unprofessional behavior. Self-regulation becomes professional group regulation of every member.

Learning from experience includes developing a constructively critical eye toward one's own and the others' behavior. Upholding group values is the responsibility of all those who participate in the profession. Collective perspective taking and self-regulation capabilities are often how high-profile professions are judged "from the outside" by the public. Nothing tarnishes the image of a profession or diminishes the public's trust more than accusations that unprofessional behaviors of individuals are "covered up" by others within the profession. In *Boston Magazine*'s February 2003 edition, a major story title read "The Silent Treatment" with the following caption:

> Boston may be a medical mecca, but it's a reputation doctors and hospitals protect so fiercely that they're keeping secret the mistakes they make. And what you don't know could hurt you. (Most, 2003, p. 105)

SELF-ASSESSMENT AND REFLECTION APPLIED TO SOCIAL BEHAVIOR

Professionalism is realized in the doctor–patient relationship through humility, commitment to competence or intellectual honesty, and the appropriate self-assessment of ability and sense of responsibility. These traits are attained through *self-assessment* to gain insight into the self's knowledge and knowledge about self—what you know and don't know and how you learn best. Included in this is how you relate to peers and supervisors and how you should respond to supervision. *Self-knowledge* includes admitting that you are the learner and that the attending is the teacher. In some instances, it may also mean that you don't know something and that you need to ask for help. Learners become experts when they *reflect* on their response to supervision and *recognize* the difference between accepting responsibility and overstepping boundaries.

In rare instances, lack of responsibility (and associated metacognitive capabilities) signifies complete perspective-taking failure. In March 2004, the lead article in the *Boston Globe* chronicled the story of a doctor caught in an infamous act of leaving the operating room with the patient on the table to cash his paycheck. This doctor subsequently engaged in a string of unprofessional and illegal behaviors. The irony was "the lingering disbelief that such a brilliant and compassionate doctor—some say the most brilliant and most compassionate they had ever known—could seem to self-destruct in such a spectacularly public way" (Swidey, 2004, p. 22).

Clues to the doctor's demise were evident in the descriptions of his behaviors offered by friends and associates. Although he was characterized as intensely compassionate with his patients, he was also depicted as self-absorbed, arrogant, narcissistic, and lacking insight when it came to relationships with others. He often confused and demeaned the coworkers around him. He lacked an appreciation of boundaries. If asked, this doctor would most likely have expressed an intense identity with the profession. However, he lacked the metacognitive capacity to regulate and control his professional behavior.

Wear and Castellani (2000) provide some insight into the "higher-order" skills needed to be professional within the doctor–patient relationship. They conclude that instead of viewing professionalism as a series of specific content areas or personality character traits, we should view it as "an ongoing, self-reflective *process* involving habits of thinking, feeling and acting" (p. 603). They propose to move away from an "ends" approach to professionalism, that is, one that defines the values, guidelines, mores, and attitudes, to an approach that focuses on means. This approach requires the development of metacognitive capabilities that will enable learners to engage in professional behavior and learn from the experiences throughout their lifetimes.

CULTURAL AWARENESS

Professionalism in the doctor–patient relationship presumes the ability to take the patient's perspective and to respect his or her values and beliefs even if they are different from one's own. Cultural awareness and sensitivity are manifestations of professionalism that demand metacognitive skill in reflection and perspective taking. At its highest level, the latter involves acceptance and respect. Berger (in Wear & Castellani, 2000) describes the "mobile mind," a metacognitive concept, as a skill set that involves respecting/embracing multiple human values and orientations—even those that are different than one's own. According to Berger, this entails a cosmopolitan way of thinking—broad-mindedness, or an openness to the environment around us, including a sensitivity to differences and respect for others (Wear & Castellani, 2000). Berger's concept of the sociologic consciousness mirrors professionalism and offers insight into the metacognitive abilities involved.

Intuition and Stereotyping

There is considerable evidence that the unconscious base of rapid cognition or intuition, an essential component of expertise, is also at the root of some unprofessional behavior. Studies have shown that unconscious behavior in certain contexts can explain unfair discrimination among individuals with different racial characteristics. For example, in a study that tightly controlled other variables, Ayres (2002) found that black men were offered the worst deals on a new car, black women the second worst, white women third worst, and white men the best even after prolonged periods of negotiation.

Professional expertise requires checking intuition by consciously applying metacognition to social situations where bias and stereotyping may occur. This involves anticipating, recognizing, and reflecting on those social situations. Monitoring social perception with vigilance in situations where rapid cognition affects decisions serves as a check on unprofessional behavior. As Gladwell (2005, p. 98) states, "Taking rapid cognition seriously—acknowledging the incredible power, for good or ill, that first impressions play in our lives—requires that we take active steps to manage and control those impressions." Social behavior may be interpreted by others as unprofessional even in situations where intentions are good and relationships established. For example, jokes and sarcasm related to differences among people, even when shared with those with whom we have a relationship, may be misinterpreted more than we predict (Savitsky & Gilovich, 2003).

RESPECT

Respect requires advanced metacognitive capabilities of self-awareness, reflection, and perspective taking. As an essential component of expertise, it can be developed over time through practice and experience. For some learners and practitioners, respect is more intuitive than for others.

Individual and collective regulation can counteract disrespect that can arise in stressful contexts such as the operating room or on the floor after sleepless nights. It is in these contexts where metacognitive monitoring can break down and give way to disparaging comments about the patient. Disrespect can manifest itself early in medical training, leaving the door open for metacognitive remediation. Consider the following account.

> Richard often conveyed disrespect for the patient in comments he made during individual interactions, small-group discussions, and large-group lectures. During his first-year clinical medicine course, he insulted an elderly volunteer by refusing to participate in an exercise that involved the elderly patient because he "wasn't interested in working with old people." During a group discussion, he also conveyed disrespect toward patients who could not adhere to therapy. He said, "Well, if the patient is a moron and doesn't want to follow my recommendation, why should they bother to come and see me? They can go see someone else." In the same discussion group, when the issue of not being able to afford medications came up, he said, "If she didn't buy two packs of cigarettes a day, she would be able to pay for her medications." The discussion group leader expressed concern about Richard's unprofessional behavior in a note: "I am troubled by the possibility that Richard will be working with patients while holding these views. Some of my discomfort is at least in part informed by prior experiences with physicians who held similar views. Not only did I see the negative effects of this on patients, but I was also offended by the actual views. I feel that they were opposite to the most critical and fundamental ideals of our profession."

Individual discussions with Richard revealed that he lacked the metacognitive capabilities to respect the patient. He failed to accurately take—or even remotely approximate—the patient's perspective and could not reflect on his own perspective and responses. He saw himself expressing his individuality and failed to see the impact of his statements on others. He needed to develop respect for others, especially in situations where his values and beliefs were different. His inability to reflect on his behavior and take and accept the perspectives of others, if unchecked, will most likely lead to unprofessional behavior as a resident and practicing physician.

HONESTY AND INTEGRITY

Being honest is often intuitive but occasionally is a metacognitive decision one makes. Dishonesty becomes a metacognitive possibility when the consequences of an honest response include negative consequences to others, such as physical harm, humiliation, fear of the unknown, or damage to one's reputation. If the consequences of an honest response include such harm, then the decision to respond dishonestly may be viewed as acceptable (if no harm to others is rendered by the dishonest response). If the dishonest response in any way harms others or has no redeeming quality, then it is viewed as unacceptable. Dishonesty is unprofessional when it results in harm, and the code of ethics of the profession includes the directive to "do no harm" and to "engender the trust of others." A dishonest response may be *self-justified* if one does not or cannot view the potential harm of that response and the potential harm to self of an honest response is amplified. Reflecting on the situation and taking the perspective of others can help one choose the best and honest response. Consider the case of a junior resident.

> The resident was participating in an interaction that involved informing a 40-year-old woman with teenagers that she was pregnant. During the interview, she informed the patient of certain "pregnancy options" but purposefully made an omission. She did not raise or discuss adoption. On questioning by faculty members after the exercise, she stated that at her hospital training site, they do not talk to patients about adoption. When a suggestion was made to discuss this with a social worker in the site, she resisted and said, "The social worker also does not talk about adoption or about pregnancy options." She said that she is specifically "told not to use certain communication styles and vocabulary including adoption." The faculty members, not being thoroughly familiar with the resident's primary training site, thought the response was unusual. Subsequent discussions by supervising faculty with the residency director and social workers in the resident's training site revealed that indeed this option is presented to patients and that the resident is well aware. Further insight into the reason for the dishonesty can be gained by understanding the resident's perspective. During subsequent discussions, she stated that she "is afraid to ask patients certain questions because they may open up certain problems that she may not be able to solve." She acknowledged that not being in control of the medical situation makes her quite uncomfortable. She did not see any harm in responding to the faculty members the way she did.

If the resident had been able to reflect in action on her own fear of lack of control and anticipate the potential harm to others (faculty, colleagues, and future patients of those faculty), she could have chosen the appropriate honest response. The stronger her metacognitive capabilities and professional identity, the more likely she would have chosen the honest response.

ALTRUISM

Altruism is the highest level of perspective taking in that it involves *seeing and valuing* the world as others see and value it. It includes the ability to recognize and surrender one's own values and motivations in order to serve the other and the "common good." Paul Farmer, MD, whose altruistic behaviors are chronicled by Tracy Kidder in *Mountains Beyond Mountains*, is referred to as a "do-gooder, in the most profound, fundamental perception of the word" (Claridge, 2003, p. D8). It is the ability to see others' views, combined with values of respect for others and selflessness, that defines the collective consciousness. Farmer responds to being called a saint: "It's not that I mind it. It's that it's inaccurate" (Kidder, 2003, p. 16).

Altruism is born from seeing things as others do and doing things for others, especially those who can least do it for themselves. It is doing the "right thing" regardless of the uphill battle or the eventual outcome. In fact, the intended outcome *is* the process. As Farmer states, "It should be enough to humbly serve the poor" (Kidder, 2003, p. 256). As a reminder that altruism is a human characteristic that stems from perspective taking and that motivation to be altruistic is incidental, Claridge (2003) describes Farmer as somewhat arrogant as well. Gaining insight into Farmer's brand of altruism, he himself states, "There's a lot to be said for sacrifice, remorse, even pity. Still the goal remains clear: 'If you don't work hard, someone will die who doesn't have to.' . . . It's what separates us from roaches" (Kidder, 2003, pp. 41, 191).

We often recognize the features of altruism by its absence. Consider the following example of the absence of altruism as described by a lamenting colleague.

> A 16-year-old patient was admitted to the intensive care unit because of status asthmaticus and decompressed respiratory acidosis and was intubated within a couple of minutes and supported with a ventilator. In the ER, the pulmonologist and the primary care physician on call were notified about the admission and the critical state of the patient. The pulmonologist rushed to the hospital and spent the next 3 to 4 hours with the patient. The responsible admitting physician managed the case by phone. The patient's family was not approached by either physician with an explanation of the critical status. The following day, the patient became worse and was transferred to a tertiary care facility. The family was upset because they had not been consulted during the night. When the admitting physician was asked by a colleague why he didn't go to the ER, he responded that there was no reason to be there if the specialist was already taking care of the patient. The colleague told him that the family probably was expecting to see him with the patient—to which he responded that he still didn't think he needed to be there. (UMMS Faculty Member, personal communication, December 11, 2003)

Did the admitting physician exhibit unprofessional behavior or poor judgment? What's clear is that he failed to see the family's perspective in relation to his own.

SUMMARY

Metacognitive capabilities applied to social, cultural, and ethical concerns constitute the foundation of professionalism. These capabilities should be applied to the self as individual or as a member of the collective medical identity. Viewing and taking the other's perspective is especially important for professional behavior. Regulating the profession is monitoring the validity of the growing body of knowledge and addressing unprofessional behavior (collective and individual). Regulating one's professional behavior is a matter of acting how others expect a member of the profession to act.

Rather than focus attention on professional content areas and behaviors such as appropriate dress or answering a page, the responsible thought processes of reflection and perspective taking should be the focus of medical education. Specifically, it is important to enhance the learner's metacognition related to the social and cultural context. As Scardamalia (2002, p. 603) states, "The development of professionalism so conceived is not fostered by lists of abstract qualities, end-of term checklists, or virtue checkpoints throughout the curriculum."

CHAPTER NINE

Teaching Expertise

INTRODUCTION

The previous chapters begin to define the content and goals of a curriculum devoted to helping medical students achieve expertise. This chapter offers specific recommendations for teaching expertise and the underlying processes of intuition and metacognition. The strategies described in this chapter cover a broad range of faculty-directed activities that engage the learner. They include (a) reflective writing and reading exercises that focus on narratives; (b) interactive teaching styles that facilitate reflection, self-assessment, and perspective-taking; (c) feedback designed to improve self-assessment as well as performance; and (d) modeling metacognition. These strategies are brought to life with examples from colleagues and from the literature.

TEACHING STRATEGIES

Medical school faculty can foster the development of medical expertise by enabling their students to develop intuitive and metacognitive capabilities through planning, modeling, choosing the appropriate teaching style, and providing feedback. They can help learners be vigilant about observing and interpreting their own and others' behaviors, thoughts, and feelings within a rigorous training program that focuses on experience gained in clinical practice. Specifically, the medical teacher can adopt the following strategies:

1. Foster reflective writing and reading. Teaching from text is a rich tradition in medical education. Books, journal articles, and handouts provide the cognitive foundation for basic science and

clinical medicine. A special genre of text—one that relates to both narratives and scripts—can be used to teach metacognition.

2. Use a facilitative teaching style that includes reflective questioning. The teacher's interaction with learners is perhaps the most prevalent and powerful means of teaching metacognition. Teaching styles represent the range of verbal and nonverbal behaviors that teachers use during interactions with their students. Some styles are oriented toward cognitive growth, such as providing information and comparing and contrasting concepts and ideas. The facilitative style can be used to probe metacognition or thoughts about thinking and feeling.

3. Provide feedback on thinking, perspective taking, and reflection. Feedback should more often be directed at how one thinks and feels compared to how others think and feel and what one thinks about his or her thoughts and feelings.

4. Model reflection, self-assessment, and self-evaluation. Finally, modeling or demonstrating behavior can be used to teach metacognitive capabilities. It is a particularly powerful way of teaching in the presence of the patient. It can help teach metacognition if it engages the learner's thought process before, during, and after the demonstration.

TEACHING FROM TEXT

Experiential Narratives

Students can learn from experience and apply metacognitive and intuitive thinking through reading and/or writing narratives. Narratives focus on the reflections of self and others. They provide an opportunity to understand others' perspectives on a shared (i.e., common) experience. Narratives can be used to learn about the physician–patient relationship and medical problem solving. Kleinman (1988, p. xiv) states, "It is clinically useful to learn how to interpret the patient's and family's perspective on illness. Indeed, the interpretation of narratives of illness experience, I will argue, is a core task in the work of doctoring, although the skill has atrophied in biomedical training." The use of narrative is an extremely powerful method of sharing reflections on *experience* within the one-to-one teaching interaction or with groups of learners and professionals.

The experience shared in a narrative may focus on a chain of events or reflections about the meaning of events. One seminal event—the critical incident—may also serve as a central theme for an experiential narrative. The *critical incident* as a focus for reflection has been discussed elsewhere in the literature (Brookfield, 1995). Writing and collecting experiential narratives can enhance the medical school curriculum and facilitate lifelong learning. As Borkan, Reis, and Medalie (2001, p. 129) state, "Collecting and recording such stories (rarely done in busy practices) allows us to organize our experiences and reflect back on our patients and our own actions and life-courses."

Experiential narratives can focus the reader's reflections on any combination of perspectives—those of the patient, the family, or the provider(s). They can be used to analyze a patient's perspective on illness (i.e., the experience of disease) or to contrast the patient's perspective with that of another patient, family member, or doctor. They can also describe a physician's or student's reflections about his or her own or the patient's thoughts and feelings. The layers of perspectives and reflections that constitute the meaning of an experience are illuminated by the experiential narrative.

Experiential narratives can be in-depth accounts of personal experiences. Biographies, autobiographies, and nonfiction reports of physician experiences that are rich with experiential accounts and/or metacognitive reflections abound (e.g., Williams, 1984). They can also be short personal reflections that powerfully dissect human experience on multiple levels. These shorter experiential narratives can focus on a single metacognitive lesson (e.g., comparing your view of sexuality with an adolescent's) and can be culled from the literature or created and cataloged locally for teaching purposes. Often their creation can serve multiple goals (e.g., to develop faculty *and* to model reflection for students).

Consider the following experienced physician's recollection of a 7-year-old girl who was *his patient* many years ago during medical school (Kleinman, 1988). This very brief written narrative excerpted from the literature focuses on the value of eliciting oral illness narrative from patients. It demonstrates the immense and long-lasting value of both written and oral narratives for patients, practicing physicians, and learners. The narrative presents a metacognitive analysis of the experience reflecting on each day the patient underwent the excruciating surgical ritual of debridement, which was an ordeal for the *hand-holding* medical student as well as the patient:

> I could barely tolerate the daily horror: her screams, dead tissue floating in the blood-stained water [of the whirlpool] the peeling flesh, the oozing wounds, the battles over cleaning and bandaging. Then one day, I made contact. At wit's end, angered at my own ignorance and impotence, uncertain what to do besides clutching the small hand, and in despair over her unrelenting anguish, I found myself asking her to tell me how she tolerated it, what the feeling was like of being so badly burned and having to experience the awful surgical ritual, day after day. She stopped, quite surprised, and looked at me from a face so disfigured it was difficult to read the expression; then in terms direct and simple, she told me. While she spoke, she grasped my hand harder

and neither screamed nor fought off the surgeon or the nurse. Each day from then on, her trust established, she tried to give me a feeling of what she was experiencing. (Kleinman, 1988, pp. xi–xii)

Teaching about the doctor–patient relationship is particularly challenging. Engaging students in the lessons learned from "real-time" life experiences can be a *hit-or-miss* proposition. Experiential narratives uniquely capture the relational, emotional, and evaluative elements of the experience of doctoring in a format that transcends time and space. They document the experience of relationship—the thoughts and feelings about thoughts and feelings—and transform the experience into learning potential.

The following experiential narrative written by a colleague addresses several key features of the physician–patient relationship. Consider how it can be used with learners to facilitate reflection about culture, time, observation, caring, relating, and regret.

> Good bye, Senor Rosario. Your last days of dying and your death came somewhat suddenly, while I was away at a conference. Your lungs wore out, filling with fluid and fibrosis in some mysterious combination, and your grieving family surrounded your intensive care bed, carefully considered your previous wishes, and chose comfort over continued ventilation.
>
> Two evenings later, I, the agnostic Anglo doctora, hurried back into the city for the last few minutes of your wake, trying not to miss that. Even the funeral home entrance was crowded, but your daughter saw me walk in and came to greet me. We spoke of your last days; she wondered as all families do in the immediacy of grief, if she had talked you into coming to the office or the hospital sooner, would it have made a difference? She directed me to the viewing room to find your wife.
>
> I followed the musical sound of Spanish praying, eventually realizing it was the rosary, into the room with your casket, and felt the low mumble of the crowds of family and friends, saw a few of my patients who must have known you in this obviously close-knit, small-city Latino community. At the back of the hall, waiting to greet your wife, I watched and listened and learned more about you than I'd ever known. In your death I have finally learned of the life you lived.
>
> In all the too-short overbooked office visits of caring for you in the last half-dozen years, juggling in Spanish your multi-system medical issues—atrial fibrillation, diverticulitis, prostate cancer, renal insufficiency, now pulmonary fibrosis—I am so sorry I never got to more of these details of who you really were. I knew some of it—estranged from your wife, yet still supported by her; a still-unmarried daughter devoted to your care and very aware of all your medical needs; your own stoicism and stubbornness, your occasional frustrations with our sometimes chaotic community health center. But in this crowded wake I saw you lying peacefully amidst your large extended family, saw the

sons and daughters-in-law embracing the grieving friends, watched the grandchildren sleeping in parents' arms or entangled behind parents' coats during long hugs of sympathy. In this crowded wake I saw your real genogram, and wished so intensely that I'd known it before now, known it in time to understand it during your lived life, not your departed one.

Good-bye, Senor Rosario. I always thought that what I'd learned from caring for you was about prothrombin levels and radiation proctitis and pacemakers, but tonight I know that what I've learned from you is how much I need to put all of that into a much larger picture, how much I need to go to my patients' wakes, and how certain I am that when I go to the next one, I must already know the life, the lived genogram. (Shields, 2005)

Students and faculty can practice the *art of narrative* during their medical school courses and clerkships. They can create their own narratives, elicit those of their patients, and/or reflect on those of others. The process of developing the art of narrative can begin by having medical students in their longitudinal preceptorships elicit and reflect on patients' stories. Kleinman (1988, p. 256) states, "Skill in mini-ethnography can be honed by sending students out of the lecture hall and hospital to follow up on their patients in the local community. They can observe patients at home and in their dealings with health care and social welfare agents and agencies." As students gain experience in eliciting the illness narratives, they can add their reflections about their own and others' thoughts and feelings. They can share their experiential narratives with other learners and faculty members. They can read the narratives of experts and add their own reflections. Through reflection, stories that document experience become experiential narratives that promote metacognition.

Experiential narratives prepared by learners can be used effectively as self-directed learning exercises or combined with other teaching methods to promote individual or group learning. At the individual level, a preceptor can review a student's narrative and share his or her thoughts about the student's reflections with that student. The narrative can also be used in small-group discussions where students can view multiple perspectives. The practice of sharing experiential narratives breaks down traditional barriers in medicine and medical school curricula and creates a culture of transparency (Fraser & Greenhalgh, 2001; Pringle, Bradley, Carmichael, Wallis, & Moore, 1995).

Metacognitive Scripts

Scripts have gained attention as methods of documenting the way *expert physicians* think about, explain, and solve clinical problems on the basis of experience. They can take many forms and be used throughout the

curriculum to teach clinical problem solving. For example, early in medical school, preclinical students can generate scripts to demonstrate cognitive understanding of the basic science of medicine. Early learners or
novices will present scripts that are disorganized and focused on anatomic
and pathophysiologic features and explanations (Abernathy & Hamm,
1995). Expert physicians, on the other hand, will tend to use contextual
features (of the patient in relation to the environment) to enhance pathophysiologic knowledge in clinical problem solving (Feltovich & Barrows,
1984). Klein (1998) suggests that scripts are a superb method of teaching about complex cases that have many metacognitive features. Because
they capture the essence of expert decision making in complex situations,
they are considered by many to be valuable instruments for teaching intuition (Abernathy & Hamm, 1995; Abernathy & Harken, 1991).

Scripts are "trigger cases" that experts carry in their minds to expe-
dite clinical problem solving. Components of a typical script include
(a) enabling conditions (e.g., personal characteristics, such as a 35-
year-old with IV drug use); (b) fault (e.g., sepsis, causative agent—
staphylococcus); and (c) consequences (acute heart condition, fever, ane-
mia, and weight loss = endocarditis) (Schmidt, Norman, & Boshuizen,
1990). During the course of clinical practice, physicians *mentally collect*
scripts, then search their collections for matching characteristics during
subsequent problem-solving encounters. According to Abernathy and
Hamm (1995, p. 334), "The value of scripts is based upon two features
of the human mind: (a) its ability to construct large mental structures
that can act as a unit and (b) its ability to recognize things rapidly. Scripts
enable experts to take advantage of the mind's strengths so that they can
handle all situations in their domain of expertise."

Scripts can pose a danger to clinical outcomes if they are not validated
through reflection or evidence-based review. They become *metacognitive
scripts* only when they include *reflections about the problem-solving process in relation to the outcomes.* One expert physician described reflection about the problem-solving process as being "like a voice in my head
asking me if this patient's health may be more significantly at risk . . . the
IGBO (I got burned once) principle. That is to say, this case of hematuria
in front of me looks a lot like the other guy I saw last year and I missed
his bladder cancer. I find this voice is stronger than the collective voice
of the many patients with hematuria." Self-questioning is an important
skill in the creation of metacognitive scripts and is discussed further in
chapter 10.

The differences between novice and expert scripts lie not only in the
problem solutions but also in the organization of knowledge and the characteristics of the thinking itself (Abernathy & Hamm, 1995). Advanced students and experts will generate scripts that exemplify greater metacognitive

characteristics—*reflective and organizational features*—than their novice counterparts. The premise underlying the metacognitive script is that the physician preparing to meet with the patient must initially *activate* a script and then *observe and reflect* on his or her experience with the patient.

Narrative reflection of underlying assumptions, motivations, thoughts, and feelings interwoven with cognitive features such as enabling conditions, fault, and consequences elucidate the clinical problem-solving process. The metacognitive script includes reflections about problem solving and is particularly illustrative of the complexity of patient care decisions that are made in the context of teams that include students and residents. In those contexts, *intuition* of expert faculty is based on greater experience with both patients and learners. The metacognitive script includes the *case* with personal reflections and a *discussion* that can include the perspectives of several reviewers, each focusing on his or her own thoughts and feelings.

The following account of a surgeon's approach to an 88-year-old woman with vague abdominal pain is adapted to highlight metacognitive processes from Abernathy and Hamm (1995, p. 170). The case description presents the surgeon's thinking and reflections about the case. A discussion has been added as a metacognitive review.

Surgical Case Description

[According to the referring doctor,] she has a tender mobile mass in her abdomen that he thought was 2 or 3 inches in size. "My first immediate thought is, she's going to need an operation." A first issue is whether the colon is involved: "I don't want to just barge into an operation where there are pitfalls and traps to fall into, such as operating on an un-prepped colon if it were a colonic mass and then having to give a colostomy." The referring doctor said that he did a pelvic examination and that it was not gynecologic; thus the mass could be in the colon.

The patient is admitted to the hospital. The surgeon reads the referring letter, which has basically the same information. The surgeon visits the patient's bedside.

History. The patient is depressed and senile, not a reliable source of history: "The history was basically worthless, except that she was eating, she was moving her bowels. She wasn't having very much pain. So that told me a lot of things it wasn't—it's not appendicitis."

Physical Examination. The surgeon does a pelvic examination and feels a mobile mass in the area of the uterus. "I do not think it's bowel. How can the bowel be that big without blocking it? She's been eating, she doesn't have a fever, she's got some pain. So she's got a big fibroid uterus, or else she's got a malignancy in her uterus.

Operation. Upon operation an ovarian cyst the size of a fist is discovered and removed.

Discussion and Metacognitive Analysis

This script provides a detailed account of the problem-solving process and the surgeon's thoughts. In this script there is evidence of intuition and metacognition underlying expert judgment at many junctures. Without all of the evidence in hand, and with "questionable" or even "suspect" information from the patient and referring physician, the surgeon makes a fairly quick decision to operate. He does so relying on pattern recognition. Rather than focus on confirming the diagnosis, which is unnecessary, he is already thinking ahead to the operation; trying to avoid "pitfalls," such as an un-prepped colon if the problem is colon cancer.

Novice or inexperienced surgeons would likely hesitate to "move on the case" without confirmatory data. The surgeon's thought to himself, "She's going to need an operation," was sufficient for triggering the next step—have the gynecologist perform the operation. The operation itself became a diagnostic tool and, in turn, produced important information. As Abernathy and Hamm (1995, p. 171) state, "Only at surgery was the problem specifically identified as an ovarian tumor and the specific action (removal) decided. . . . It is interesting that the expert's reasoning was 'only as precise as it needed to be.' There was no call for expensive, unneeded diagnostic procedures such as CT or MRI that may have been ordered by more novice clinicians."

Metacognitive scripts can be used to achieve many specific objectives related to problem solving. One objective is to enable students to define the impact of different physician perspectives on problem solving. This is accomplished by having expert faculty from different specialties write the discussion of the metacognitive script. Students can read the cases and discussions and compare the thought processes of physicians from different specialties (e.g., primary care or surgery) or with different personal characteristics (e.g., gender or culture).

Experiential narratives and metacognitive scripts can be used to develop faculty and teach learners in a number of contexts. Faculty members develop greater insight into their thinking processes and sharpen their reflective capabilities, hallmarks of effective teaching and practice (Brookfield, 1995). A metacognitive script library could be established from which faculty members could draw material to learn from each other as well as to teach to specific learner objectives.

INTERACTING WITH THE LEARNER

Role Play

Role play is an opportunity for learners to develop metacognitive capabilities, such as perspective taking, in a secure environment. Typically, students interview simulated patients (standardized or peers) during clinical case scenarios. Klein (1998, p. 42) suggests that simulation is the preferred method of teaching "more difficult cases." From a curricular point of view, it would be advantageous to develop a series of role-play exercises that represent progressively more specific complex cases within certain genres, such as *managing chronic illness in children* or *motivational and lifestyle counseling with adolescents*. Students could chronicle their participation and progress on developing their capabilities in each series and reflect on their learning experiences. They would learn to assess needs, take perspectives, monitor performance, and plan educational experiences.

Role-play exercises promote perspective taking, reflection, and self-assessment. The problem-oriented interview with a simulated patient is only one example of role play to develop metacognition. There are many variations that can be used in the actual clinical teaching encounter as well. Brief role-taking exercises can address specific learning objectives after a patient interaction. For example, the preceptor can simply ask the learner *to step into the shoes of the patient:* "What would you think if you were the teenage patient you just interviewed and I asked you—Are you sexually active?" and then "How else could you get the information in a way that would lessen the risk of embarrassing the patient?" This same strategy could be used in preparation for a learner–patient interaction. The student not only learns to look at the meaning of words from another view but also learns to predict and anticipate the impact of words before they are presented. The more often the learner is challenged to take the perspective of the patient (or nurse, consultant, and so on) and discuss it with the preceptor or attending, the more reliable he or she will become at perspective taking. Using the predicted patient's perspective to check for actual perspective or to act (e.g., provide patient education or empathize) should improve clinical performance and outcomes.

A variation of this exercise is to have the teacher take the role of the patient and have the student play him- or herself. The ensuing discussion can include reflection by both the learner and the teacher (patient). The goal here is to enable the learner to explore anticipated or experienced thoughts and feelings in a "safe" environment. The student can learn about potential patient responses from one who is experienced and adapt his or her behaviors accordingly. When time permits, students can reflect on these role-taking experiences in writing. An adaptation of this method has been explored in the world of business education. Argyris (1989) describes having two learners engage in a conversation that is recorded and transcribed. The transcripts are then given to each individual to make notes about "what you meant" and about "what you thought the other person meant." The notes (i.e., reflections on perspective) are then shared.

Teaching Style

Teaching metacognition relies heavily on the quality of interactions between the teacher and the learner. Generally, the teacher is the attending or preceptor, although it could also be a resident or peer who teaches the student. In these interactions, the teacher can choose the appropriate teaching behaviors that facilitate metacognition and intuition. Teaching behaviors can be grouped into styles that reflect the emphasis placed on the learner's role in the learning process. A more complete discussion of teaching styles can be found in an earlier book (Quirk, 1994).

Each of four teaching styles is appropriate for achieving a specific level of objectives or for addressing a type of capability. Figure 9.1 illustrates the relationship between metacognition and teaching styles. Figure 9.2 presents specific teaching behaviors associated with each style.

As the figures suggest, assertive and suggestive teaching styles are most appropriate for helping the learner develop a cognitive base (i.e., gain knowledge and understanding). They are teacher directed, information or opinion oriented, and geared toward assessing and expanding the learner's knowledge base and ability to apply that knowledge. The facilitative and collaborative teaching styles, on the other hand, encourage the development of metacognitive capabilities, including reflection, self-questioning, perspective taking, and self-assessment. Open-ended

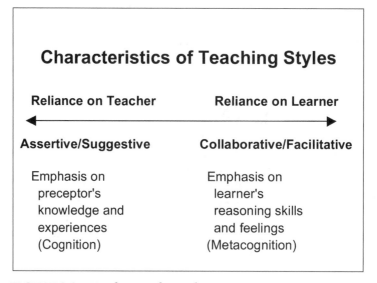

FIGURE 9.1   Teaching styles and metacognition

Assertive	Suggestive	Collaborative	Facilitative
Gives directions	Suggests alternatives/ choices	Elicits/accepts learner's ideas	Elicits/accepts learner's feelings
Asks focused questions	Asks leading questions	Uses open/explorat- ory questions	Uses open/reflective questions
Gives information	Gives opinions	Relates personal experiences	Offers feelings encouragement

FIGURE 9.2   Teaching styles and related behaviors

and reflective questioning and relating personal experience are important facilitative teaching behaviors. Consider the following two teaching vignettes. In the first example, the teacher focuses on cognition; in the second, he facilitates self-reflection and perspective taking using a facilitative style.

Vignette 1: Assertive Style; Focus on Cognition

STUDENT: Do you have a few minutes . . . can I tell you about a patient I am seeing?

PRECEPTOR: Sure, why don't you present her to me?

STUDENT: OK, she's a 15-year-old girl who came in for a physical. I've seen her before for an ear infection, and she came in with her mom with a form she needs filled out, and I'm just not really sure what I should be doing on a physical for a 15-year-old.

PRECEPTOR: What kind of reasons would you want to do a physical on a 15-year-old?

STUDENT: Well, I've seen a bunch of well-child checks, and done physicals on some of my elderly patients, but 15-year-olds I haven't seen very much, and they don't come in for physicals very often.

PRECEPTOR: This is a common problem, but they come in more than you think. They may have a form to be filled out for camp or for school or for work or to get their immunizations updated, or they may be having a specific problem; sometimes they're having menstrual problems. Did you take a menstrual history?

STUDENT: No, I didn't even really think about that.

PRECEPTOR: OK, well, that's an important thing, and you ought not skip over that because that leads up to whether or not a 15-year-old needs to have a pelvic exam. Did you do a pelvic exam?

STUDENT: No, I did not even think about that either.

PRECEPTOR: OK, well, that's an important thing to think about. There may be a number of reasons that you may want to do a pelvic exam. Do you know what those might be?

STUDENT: Umm . . . do you do pelvics on all the 15-year-olds you see?

PRECEPTOR: No, absolutely not, that depends from the menstrual history, whether she's sexually active, or whether she is at risk for an STD, or whether she is having any kind of problems. And this gets complicated even more by the way the room is set up. Is her mother in there with her?

STUDENT: Yeah, she is, and I am not sure I can even ask her some of the questions that you are talking about with her mom in the room— I mean she would be really uncomfortable.

PRECEPTOR: Well, I'll tell you what. She is still in the room right now, and we are sort of running out of time. Why don't we go in together, and I'll take the history and show you how I handle both the history taking and dealing with the mother in the room. And then we can step out and I can tell you what I think about whether or not she needs to have a pelvic exam done. OK?

STUDENT: OK, that will be good.

Vignette 2. Facilitative Style; Focus on Metacognition

STUDENT: Do you have a few minutes. . . . Can I tell you about a patient I'm seeing?

PRECEPTOR: Sure (silence).

STUDENT: It's Betty Wood, she's a 15-year-old, and she came in with a form for a physical to be filled out. I mean, when I look through the chart, I've seen her for otitis media and follow her dad for hypertension. When I went through her exam, I listened to her heart, listened to her lungs, felt her abdomen, but I wasn't sure if there was anything else I should be focusing on.

PRECEPTOR: What do you think is important to cover?

STUDENT: Now that I think about it, I may want to pay attention to things like menstrual history and cigarettes and drugs; you know, sexuality and things like that.

PRECEPTOR: That's good. That's all important stuff. It sounds like you may not have covered all that with her.

STUDENT: Yeah, you know I guess I'm thinking adolescence kind of sums up this whole thing, and that just seems like a tough issue.

PRECEPTOR: Yeah, what makes that tough for you?

STUDENT: Well, she was pretty uncomfortable, and she seemed pretty nervous about doing this, so I guess I just did the history and physical, filled out the form, and just left it at that.

PRECEPTOR: Yeah, well, it's important to pay attention to her level of discomfort; what about your own?

STUDENT: Oh . . . I guess . . . I mean she's 15, but she's pretty developed sexually. I mean I am not that much older than her, and I was pretty uncomfortable there too. I wasn't quite sure how to bring up some of these topics, especially with my own discomfort.

PRECEPTOR: Yeah, it's great that you recognize that these are powerful feelings and that they influence the interaction. They happen to all of us, they happen to me, and some of them get better with experience. For instance, can you think of some ways that you might be able to approach taking that kind of history that would make it more comfortable for you and for her?

STUDENT: You know, maybe things like asking about menstrual history first. That seems a little bit less threatening and maybe telling her that there are a few things that may be uncomfortable but I talk about with every new patient that I see. Might make it more comfortable both for me and for her.

PRECEPTOR: Well, I'll tell you what. She is still in the room right now, and we are sort of running out of time. Why don't we go in together; I'll ask the mother to leave the room, and you'll take the history. And then we can step out and discuss whether or not she needs to have a pelvic exam done. OK?

STUDENT: OK, that will be good.

The preceptor in the first interaction is the "sage on the stage" and in the second is the "guide on the side" (Fraser & Greenhalgh, 2001, p. 803). The differences between the two interactions are evident in who is doing the talking. In the first interaction, the preceptor predominantly asks the learner direct questions to assess the learner's cognitive base and provides information where he feels it is necessary. Focused questions such as "What are the reasons you would want to do a physical on a 15-year-old?" are part of the assertive style. The teacher generally knows the right or wrong answers to assertive questions. The facilitative teaching style is a choice the teacher makes to enable the learner to openly think about his or her thoughts and feelings. Open questions such as "What do you think is important to cover?" and "It is important to pay attention to the patient's level of discomfort, but what about your own?" can be answered correctly only by the learner. These questions enable learners to think about their thoughts and feelings and set the stage for using and refining metacognitive capabilities.

Effective feedback is a component of teaching style and has been discussed in the literature as an essential element of medical teaching and learning (Ende, 1983). It can be provided along with information and direction as part of the assertive teaching style. For example, in vignette 1, the preceptor states, "OK, well, that's an important thing, and you ought not skip over that because that leads up to whether or not a 15-year-old needs to have a pelvic exam." Feedback can also be an important means of enhancing and reinforcing the metacognitive capabilities of reflection and self-assessment. This is evident in the feedback offered along with the preceptor's own experience (feelings) in vignette 2: "Yeah, it's great that you recognize that these are powerful feelings and that they influence the interaction. They happen to all of us, they happen to me, and some of them get better with experience."

Ideally, feedback to enhance metacognition should be preceded with questions such as "How do you think it went?" and should include open questions to promote reflection: "What do you think you could have done differently?" Other questions specifically targeting aspects of the experience such as "What were you thinking when you (or the patient) said . . . ?" and "How did you feel when she said . . . ?" can be used to promote reflection. At the end of a feedback encounter, the student could summarize and respond to the feedback. This conveys that he or she was listening and processing and attaching value to what was said.

Questions can enhance feedback by eliciting thoughts about thinking. Feedback can then focus on thinking in addition to observed performance. Consider the following questions: "What were you looking for when you asked her how her relationship with her husband is going?" "How did your feelings affect the way you responded to her anger?" Including questions in the feedback process will increase the metacognitive learning that takes place.

Modeling

Effective modeling enhances the learner's metacognitive skills. Specifically, they learn to predict and anticipate what they will see, observe and reflect on what they are seeing, and, after the experience, evaluate the process in relation to the outcomes. In essence, it is bringing the typically intuitive or unconscious aspects of experience to the consciousness level so that metacognitive learning can take place.

Modeling can be used to foster thinking about a number of aspects of doctoring. This can include interacting with the patient (history taking, educating, examining, or developing a relationship) or other providers (e.g., consultants or team members). If done effectively, modeling can provide the learner with a picture of desired behavior that can generalize to multiple contexts.

POSE is a helpful mnemonic for recalling the steps of modeling. The first step is to *preview* the interaction with the learner. Although not always an option, it enables the learner to develop the skill of anticipating what he or she will see and be able to think about possible ways to react. During preview, the teacher can help the learner identify and name issues that may come up in the impending experience and define learning objectives. In essence, the expert can help the learner frame the learning experience.

During the modeling encounter, the teacher should *outline* what he or she is doing, experiencing, and thinking. This gives the learner an opportunity to reflect on the underlying thoughts and feelings that influence the physician's decisions and behaviors. The findings that are evident to the physician during the course of the interaction should be *shared* if they are relevant and the setting is appropriate. Learners often miss connections because they are not privy to information collected by the preceptor (e.g., physical findings or information on the chart).

Finally, learners should be invited to *evaluate* the experience after it has taken place. This should include candid review of the physician's behaviors, thoughts, and feelings during and after the encounter. The following account of a modeling encounter illustrates its potential value in teaching metacognition.

Dan is a patient who was seen 6 months ago for a follow-up of abnormal liver function tests during an evaluation for diarrhea and gastritis. During the evaluation, liver function tests (LFTs) were obtained that were mildly abnormal in a pattern suggestive of nonspecific hepatitis (elevated AST [aspartate aminotransferase], ALT [alanine aminotransferase] both 1.5 times normal). You discussed the issue of abnormal LFTs with the patient. He had no symptoms and no significant past history, and he reported having about three to five glasses of wine per week. You recommended that he stop drinking completely. In 1 month, the LFTs were unchanged, and a viral hepatitis panel was negative.

The patient is in the waiting room 5 months later. The receptionist informs you that he is upset "that you didn't tell him he had hepatitis." We can see how the teacher may use the POSE mnemonic in this case:

P—You tell the student to review the chart and ask him why the patient might be upset. You ask what kinds of behaviors you might use to address the anger.

O—You greet the patient and find out that he is upset that another physician who treated him for a laceration reviewed his chart and mentioned that he had hepatitis. You try to help him understand his situation and apologize for not explaining the term "hepatitis" before.

S—You share with the student that you can understand why the patient is upset and your feeling that an apology is required. Note: Sharing your thoughts during modeling may or may not be appropriate in all situations and must be carefully considered in light of the patient's perspective. For example, sharing normal findings from auscultation is very different from sharing reflections about the patient's affective response.

E—After the interaction, you ask the student what he thought. He tells you that it sounded like you were "trying to justify" not using the word "hepatitis," and this seemed to upset the patient. He also says that when you finally apologized, it sounded sincere and that the patient seemed to become less angry.

Modeling is an effective way to teach learners how to use metacognitive skills to guide behavior. The approach presented here is particularly effective in complex situations when the connections between thinking, feeling, and behavior are not overtly recognized.

FACULTY DEVELOPMENT

Teachers become expert by engaging in the reflection process. Brookfield (1995, p. xiii) asserts that this takes place "when teachers discover and examine their assumptions by viewing their practice through four distinct, though interconnecting lenses . . . autobiographical, learners, colleagues and the literature." A faculty member needs to update not only his or her fund of knowledge but also his or her thinking process continuously. This requires taking the perspectives of others (including students) and assessing the foundations of his or her thinking (i.e., adequacy and breadth of knowledge and underlying assumptions).

Faculty members need to gain expertise in critically reflecting on their roles and performances as teachers. This includes analyses of their closest-held values and attitudes. Critical reflection, which according to Brookfield (1995) lies at the core of teaching expertise, focuses on the distorting potential of power often present in the role of teacher and the false assumptions about self that underlie poor teaching habits that evolve over time.

Teachers must become expert teachers to teach medical expertise. In this regard, they must learn and practice metacognition as it relates to teaching. It is a lifelong process in which interaction with peers and colleagues is essential. It may entail routinely discussing thoughts about patient cases and learner encounters with a colleague. Or, in the new paradigm, where faculty development is integrated into the culture of medical education, the discussions at the academic or community health center may be "critical conversation groups with colleagues that are respectful, inclusive and democratic" (Brookfield, 1995, p. 141). Discussion can refine teaching behaviors by fostering critical reflection on underlying assumptions that form the basis of expertise (metacognitive and intuitive practice).

Self-Directed Learning

INTRODUCTION

In the previous chapter, several teaching strategies for fostering metacognitive development were considered. Although some of those strategies could be implemented by the learner him- or herself, their effectiveness is enhanced by teacher and/or peer participation. The strategies described in this chapter depend on the student to direct much of his or her own learning. In other words, the student is required to assume greater responsibility for learning and to adapt to the learning environment. These student-centered strategies include planning and self-assessment, self-questioning, and reading for comprehension. Other strategies, such as portfolios and the review of patient's perspective (RPP), are offered.

LEARNING STRATEGIES

The aim of medical education is to enable students to learn that which is important for today and what will be important in the future. To become an expert, one must possess the requisite knowledge and skills and practice self-directed learning. The term "self-directed learning" has been used often with little explication of its meaning (Ainoda, Onishi, & Yasuda, 2005). In this book, self-directed learning is synonymous with the practice of metacognition. The self-directed learner must possess self-knowledge and regulate behavior. He or she must (a) know what needs to be learned (How much time should I devote tonight to "studying" for the pathology exam? What do I need to learn about caring for chronically ill patients? Do I know enough about atherosclerosis to shift the focus of my studying to ischemic heart disease?); (b) control the retrieval process (How confident am I in my answer to the question? What are the determinants of oxygen supply that affect ischemic heart disease?); (c) be aware of his or her learning style, the resources for learning, and how to access these resources; and (d) monitor his or her performance through reflection and effective perspective taking.

Learning in medical school involves successfully achieving three complex tasks related to self-directed learning: (a) assuming a greater share of control of the learning process, (b) gaining responsibility for patient care, and (c) adapting to a variety of learning environments. Each of these tasks demands the capability to plan for and monitor change on the basis of self-assessment, expected versus actual performance outcomes, and self-evaluation. Self-directed learners must also develop intrinsic motivation to learn and persistence in the face of failure or rejection. Understanding these tasks sheds light on the metacognitive foundation of self-directed learning and provides direction for curriculum development.

There is some evidence that students with the highest qualifications for medical school, as currently measured, are not necessarily the students most capable of self-directed learning. In this regard, studies have shown that admissions criteria for medical school do not predict students' self-directed learning behaviors during later professional life (Gunzburger, 1980). There is also evidence that self-directed learning is not promoted within the medical school curriculum. Once matriculated, students do not develop these learning skills over time, and neither the curriculum nor year of training has been shown to positively influence self-directed learning (Harvey, Rothman, & Frecker, 2003; Schmidt, 2000; Ward, Gruppen, & Regehr, 2002). In fact, a disturbing trend of decreasing self-directed learning over the 4 years of medical school has been noted. Curriculum designers must ask, Are we exposing our students to curricula that discourage self-directed learning? Despite this evidence, data suggest that students would like to have more opportunities to practice self-directed learning because of its perceived importance (Miflin, Campbell, & Price, 1999).

PLANNING AND CONTROLLING THE LEARNING PROCESS

Brookfield (1993, p. 229) states that "if self-direction means anything, it means that control over definitions, processes, and evaluations of learning rests with the people who are struggling to learn and not with external authorities." Control means participation in planning the learning experience. The learning cycle begins with an understanding of one's goals based on desired outcomes, proceeds to a systematic assessment (and definition) of one's deficits in relation to the goals, includes effective planning that leads to identification of resources and successful implementation of learning strategies, and proceeds to recognition and critical analysis of outcomes. It does not end there. Results feed back into goals, and the cycle begins again. To inculcate this cycle into the learner's educational experience, we introduce the mnemonic GNOME, which also serves as a guide to effective teaching.

Each day, class, study session, and patient care experience can be best approached with an understanding of *goals, needs, objectives, methods,* and *evaluation.* Whether the student is entering a classroom, studying on his or her own, or preparing to see a patient, a clear plan for learning is necessary for success. Knowing how to plan and execute self-directed learning extends medical education beyond the borders of medical school. Miflin, Campbell, and Price (2000, p. 306) state, "The ultimate goal is that, when school and faculty support is no longer available, experience in clinical practice will continue to motivate graduates, throughout their professional careers, to use their developed skills to evaluate their performance, identify personal learning needs, and select and evaluate appropriate resources to achieve their goals."

Goals

In a self-directed learning environment, goals are often determined by the major stakeholders. Professional societies and licensing associations translate current and future health care needs into curricular requirements and recommendations for medical school administrators and curriculum developers who in turn define the goals of education. They are broad competency areas that those with wisdom and expertise have deemed necessary to practice medicine. They are the starting point for needs assessment—the gold standard by which group and individual needs are assessed. In a self-directed learning environment, administrators should publicize goals and broadly include learners in the goal refinement process.

Needs

Self-assessment of learning needs is the most important component of self-directed learning and perhaps the most difficult to master. It is a skill that should be developed over time in medical school with assistance from expert faculty who can ensure validity by sharing their perspectives. As one author states, the ability "to recognize personal knowledge deficiencies is difficult to acquire, and the motivation to correct these may be hard to generate: this may require a long period of shared guidance" (ten Cate, Snell, Mann, & Vermunt, 2004, p. 225). A major hurdle initially is to overcome the tendency, especially by the least competent performers, to inflate self-assessments (Kruger & Dunning, 1999). Sclabassi and Woelfel (1984) found that medical students consistently overestimated and underestimated their own knowledge and skills when compared to their instructors on an anesthesiology clerkship. Other studies determined that most medical students tended to rate themselves lower than did their teachers or even their peers (Linn, Arostegui, & Zeppa, 1975). Gruppen et al. (1997) found that medical students thought they performed better on a clinical exercise and identified different areas of weakness than did standardized patients. Antonelli (1997, p. S65), in comparing second-year medical students' self-assessments of specific behaviors with standardized patients' assessments of these behaviors using a checklist, found that "the accuracy of the self-assessment of these specific skills was dismal." The authors conclude that there may be an "illusion of accuracy held by students in the self-assessment of clinical skills." If the standardized patients accurately represent the faculty perspective, then medical students must improve the validity of their self-assessments. They need to practice, and it needs to be taken seriously. The literature supports the need for improvement in student self-assessments (Gordon, 1991; Ward et al., 2002). This is especially pronounced for students in the clinical years, when evidence suggests less accuracy (Gruppen et al., 1997).

The most likely reason that learners do not have an accurate perception of their own behavior is that they have not developed the metacognitive skill through practice with accompanying accurate and unambiguous feedback. Antonelli (1997, p. S65) states, "These findings reinforce the value of feedback, particularly as it relates to student self-assessment accuracy. Accuracy in self-assessment of skills may be developed by building in continuing performance-based feedback along with practice and explicit criteria for students." Feedback will not only sharpen their self-assessment skills but also improve the learners' ability to see others' perspectives. This should help them develop a more accurate picture of how they are perceived by others. As might be expected, people tend to have inaccurate views of how others appraise their behaviors. In general, we believe that our flaws are more apparent than others actually perceive them. Savitsky and Gilovich (2003, p. 60) state, "We overestimate how negatively others will judge us because our transgressions loom larger to us than they do to others." This misperception could impact negatively on performance. For example, if one is anxious, this could be compounded by the false perception that others perceive the anxiety and its negative effects on behavior. Metacognitive understanding reduces the exaggerated effect, estimations become more valid, and associated performance is improved (Greer, 2005).

One strategy that has significant potential for improving self-assessments among medical students is the Q-sort method. It involves comparing students' self-assessments with those of expert using a ranking methodology to identify strengths and weaknesses (Ward et al., 2002). The approach has been applied to communication skills but hypothetically could be used to provide feedback on any capability.

Correctly assessing needs is the first step in improving outcomes. When needs are identified by students, they must feel empowered and have the means to address those needs. Gruppen et al. (1997) found that when students correctly self-assessed poor performance, they didn't take corrective measures. Educational interventions that provide the opportunity to compare self-assessments with the expert's (e.g., teacher or patient) perspective should help the novice gain greater reliability in the identification of learning needs. Defining objectives on the basis of those needs and choosing methods are additional steps in the planning process that students must be able to take.

Objectives

Objectives are the specific, measurable statements of desired outcome that the self-directed learner hopes to achieve through participation in learning experiences (Quirk, 1994). Their development has been considered exclusively within the domain of teachers rather than learners. Students can learn to define objectives to meet their own needs and guide their learning. They may or may not look to faculty-generated goals and objectives to facilitate this process. Miflin et al. (2000) discuss the importance of faculty-defined objectives as guides to students' self-directed learning. They can be discussed by the faculty member in consultation with the student to lay the foundation for self-assessment. Studies have shown that the availability of faculty-generated learning objectives for students does not, in fact, inhibit the development of self-direction (Blumberg & Michael, 1992).

Objectives express, in measurable terms, (a) cognitive (knowledge, use of knowledge, and skill), (b) affective (attitudes and feelings), and (c) metacognitive outcomes related to the underlying capabilities inherent in expertise. If possible, they also define the time frame for successful achievement. Cognitive objectives include verbs such as "define," "describe," "express," and "perform." Affective objectives must be written in the same way but include affective states, such as "I will be able to express my discomfort interviewing an elderly patient to my preceptor by tomorrow" or "I will be able to describe my fear examining a patient with HIV to the resident by the end of this week." Action sets that describe metacognitive outcomes include "express anticipation and reflection" and "demonstrate self-questioning and monitoring." A metacognitive objective would be "I will be able to reflect on, and evaluate the appropriateness of a diagnosis of appendicitis by the end of this clerkship."

Methods

Students, like teachers, must learn methods that strengthen metacognition, become facile in selecting those that best address specific objectives, and practice them with feedback. All metacognitive methods are for the most part self-directed by the learner but depend on others in the learning environment for development and implementation. Strategies are specific methods that can be implemented to achieve specific objectives. Those strategies described in the previous chapter (narratives, scripts, role play, and teaching styles) depend heavily on teachers for their implementation. The strategies described in this chapter are more student directed but can be implemented in concert with teacher-directed methods and depend on faculty mentorship.

Faculty members can *guide* learners in the development and adoption of these learning strategies. In this way, *shared direction* leads to self-directed learning. For example, they can (a) introduce the learner to strategies such as reading with metacomprehension, observing in the third person, and eliciting an RPP; (b) advise them when to use certain methods (only reading about the knee exam as a method of developing that skill would be inappropriate); and (c) reinforce and validate their use (e.g., explicit modeling, expecting the RPP as part of the oral presentation, and incorporating self-questioning into the feedback process). The self-directed learning methods described in this chapter can be blended with the more teacher-directed strategies described in the previous chapter (e.g., narratives and scripts) to achieve metacognitive objectives.

Evaluation

Evaluation data for self-directed learning experiences can come from many sources including patients, peers, and faculty members. In some instances, a predefined criterion (e.g., passing the end-of-third-year OSCE) will be the only summative measure. In more focused situations (e.g., conducting an appropriate review of systems with a hypertensive patient), the learner may want to have the preceptor observe his or her performance (via direct observation or through oral presentation) and provide feedback. In a self-directed learning environment, the learner is the final arbiter of evaluation results. In the educational planning cycle, the results of evaluation are used to revise goals and/or serve as a basis for self-assessment of learning needs.

Self-evaluation builds on reflection and is critical to functioning in groups (i.e., teamwork). Son and Schwartz (2002, p. 30) state, "Rememberers monitor the accuracy of their answers, reflected in their confidence judgments. Then, depending on the incentives, they can use their confidence judgments to alter which answers they will output and which they will withhold. Control is represented by the volunteering or withholding of answers."

STRATEGIES FOR SELF-DIRECTED LEARNING

Self-Questioning

In the new paradigm for medical education, students are encouraged to continuously assess their needs and define learning objectives. They then choose to attend lectures, select patient experiences, and read as necessary. As they engage in each of these steps of planning and learning, what they learn will be contingent on their abilities to ask themselves questions.

Questions can focus on the learner's knowledge about their own knowledge and skills. For example, before their exam, they can ask themselves, "What do I already know about hemoglobin syntheses *that I don't need to study*, and what questions about different kinds of hemoglobin will most likely appear on the test?" or "Where are the gaps in my reading?" Self-questioning can include questions about what one might learn from clinical experience: "What can I expect to learn from this diabetic patient and her family if I ask the right questions?" and "How is this experience with this adolescent patient going to be similar and different from other juvenile diabetic patients I have seen?"

On another level, self-directed questioning can look for patterns or similarities if specific previous experience is absent. For example, if the learner has not had direct experience with a diabetic patient, she can ask herself, "How is this experience with this juvenile diabetic patient going to be similar and different from the patients with juvenile rheumatoid arthritis that I have seen?" Generalizing learning through self-questioning is an essential metacognitive task related to needs assessment *in anticipation* of a learning experience.

Self-questioning knowledge and experience is a critical learning strategy for regulating behavior *in action* as well. As students interact (i.e., create new experiences) with peers, faculty, and patients, they should be encouraged to monitor the ongoing experience through self-questioning. For example, during chart rounds, the student can ask, "Where are the gaps in my knowledge base about management of juvenile diabetes as evident in what team members (residents, students, and attendings) are expressing that they know?" In the interaction with the patient that focuses on prevention of complications of diabetes, such as acidosis, shock, and coma, the student can ask him- or herself, "Am I confident that what I am saying is still valid?" and should ask as he or she educates the patient, "Am I conveying the information to the patient in a nonalarming way?"

Self-questioning is a critical component of clinical expertise. This strategy is often used by the expert clinician, before, during, and after an encounter to improve patient care. The following account of the importance of self-questioning as a check on intuition was expressed by an experienced primary care physician.

> There are many times when patients present with complaints/problems that are vague and of longish duration. No real start time, and symptoms present a lot of the time. They are often troubled by the impact the problem is having on their daily functioning, or a family member has called their attention to what is going on. Insight into what is happening can be good or quite poor. In either case, my gut/my intuition coupled with experience tells me that what is happening is in the realm of mental health. Then the dual conversation begins in my head. "Is the patient ready to hear what I am really thinking is going on?" "What do I not want to miss?" "What needs to be ruled out today?" "How much of a medical work-up will I need to do here?" "Is this patient going to get better?" This is happening inside my head while I continue to data gather and talk with the patient. At some point, it all adds up, kind of like that Far Side cartoon when a group of scientists are standing at a blackboard staring at an equation. There are a bunch of numbers and lines leading to an arrow above which says "Then a Miracle Happens," followed by an equals sign and the answer.

Self-questioning can generate important information about how to learn as well as what one knows and needs to know. How one learns depends on learning style, as described in chapter 3. Medical educators continue to call for practicing physicians to have a greater understanding of the way they learn. Greater self-understanding should result in more effective self-directed learning (e.g., uncovering the need for intrinsic motivation to learn; cf. Brookfield, 1981; Reynolds, 1986). For this reason, it is incumbent on learners to continuously refine their understanding of their learning style through self-questioning during the learning experience (Airey, Marriott, & Rodd, 2001).

Reading for Comprehension

Medical faculty can help students develop self-assessment skills related to comprehension that will benefit their learning throughout their professional lives. Students can be taught to monitor what they learn from text in relation to predefined goals. Faculty at the University of Kansas have developed a model of strategy instruction that has been effective in helping learners develop self-directed learning skills related to reading comprehension. A core group of strategies advocated by the Kansas group include self-questioning, visual imagery, mnemonics, and error analysis (Deshler & Schumaker, 1988). These and other recommended reading strategies require a level of metacognitive sophistication that is not often considered in medical education. Pressley (2002, p. 304) describes the metacognitively sophisticated reader as

> knowing that comprehension is most likely by reading actively; that is, the good reader knows to relate what is being read to prior knowledge, and he or she is aware that good readers predict what might be in upcoming text and relate ideas encountered in text to their prior knowledge. The metacognitively sophisticated reader also knows to ask questions while reading, construct images of ideas being conveyed in text, and summarize what is being read. The metacognitively sophisticated reader knows that good reading involves being alert to the possibility that some parts of the text are confusing. He or she knows to react to confusion with fix-up strategies, such as rereading. The metacognitively sophisticated reader knows comprehension strategies, knows to use them and often does use them.

Before reading, good readers have a plan that includes understanding the goals of reading (How much do I have to get done, and for what reason?) and the time frame involved. Effective readers tend to activate prior knowledge and relate current reading to that knowledge. Pressley proposes that good readers also tend to be evaluative of the text they are reading (Is it credible and trustworthy?), and they monitor what they read (Is it relevant to my goals, and how are the sections related to the whole?). They also constantly ask themselves, What am I getting out of this, and what am I not understanding? After the first reading, the metacognitive reader reflects on what was gained and what was missed and may even reread to gain better comprehension. As Pressley (2002, p. 298) states, "There has been much experimental evidence establishing that when readers are taught to use comprehension strategies, their comprehension improves."

Studies demonstrate that college students who perform poorly also tend to be poor monitors of their comprehension. They are overconfident in their predictions about test performance relative to good performers (Maki & McGuire, 2002). On the other hand, top students tend to be most capable of monitoring and improving their comprehension. This is the capability of metacomprehension (Maki & Berry, 1984). One would expect that medical students who are top performers in their classes would be most capable in this area. However, faculty members must play an active role in selecting text at the correct level for their learners. Texts of medium difficulty, relative to low or high difficulty, tend to be correlated to the highest level of metacomprehension (Weaver & Bryant, 1995). The evidence also suggests that self-monitoring of comprehension is most likely when the difficulty level of the text is matched to the reader's capability (Maki & McGuire, 2002). Faculty members and other learning resources can help learners assess their reading levels, provide readings at the appropriate levels, and encourage learners to monitor their comprehension as they read.

There is some evidence that metacognition is an important factor, perhaps even a prerequisite for reading comprehension. The authors of one study conclude that students must be able to recognize the need and then monitor the opportunities to connect concepts in order to comprehend what they read (Britton, Stimson, Stennett, & Gulgoz, 1998). Metacognition supports the mechanical and cognitive components of reading by motivating and enabling the activation of prior learning. Metacognitive monitoring can thus be viewed as a "triggering variable" for reading comprehension (Maki & McGuire, 2002, p. 62). Metacomprehension can be introduced early through workshops and seminars and reinforced throughout medical school.

The curriculum and faculty should (a) emphasize and model the importance of making connections (especially across disciplinary boundaries), (b) choose reading material that reinforces connections and is appropriate for the students' levels, and (c) reinforce the need to connect the concepts during reading. Strategies might include discussion questions, pop quizzes, portfolios, and other writing assignments that document the connections that students are making and their monitoring behaviors. The monitoring behaviors would include defining realistic goals for reading within the allotted time, skimming before reading, attending to headings, and rereading when necessary. Developing and reinforcing metacognitive strategies should improve comprehension now and in the learner's future. Pressley (2002, p. 291) states, "Long-term instruction of sophisticated comprehension strategies clearly improves student understanding and memory of texts that are read." There is evidence that many college and medical students would benefit from such metacognitive reading instruction (Pressley, 2002; Quirk, 1994; Simpson & Nist, 2002).

Reading comprehension strategies should focus on the elements of active reading, such as predicting, questioning, imaging, clarifying, and summarizing while reading (Pressley, 2002). For example, rather than simply assigning a handout to be read, faculty members could instruct learners to first write a paragraph predicting the important points to be made and, at the end, a final paragraph comparing the prediction to postanalysis. The assignment could also include a list of important self-questions asked during active reading. Incorporating these strategies into the curriculum alongside methods of teaching cognition, teachers can become active facilitators of metacomprehension.

Learning Portfolios

The learning portfolio has great potential as both a self-directed learning strategy and an evaluation instrument. It provides an opportunity for metacognitive analyses of one's own performance related to many different competencies or capabilities. It has many advantages over traditional learning and self-evaluation methods. It is "asynchronous" and can be adapted to a Web-based format for ease of sharing (Carraccio & Englander, 2004). Some medical educators suggest that it keeps individuals interested and engaged in their own individual learning processes (Airey et al., 2001). It has great potential for monitoring and regulating learning throughout a lifetime.

Portfolios include data that enhance metacognitive growth and development. Medical students, residents, and practicing physicians alike may construct portfolios that include learning needs, practice goals and expectations, and the metrics to demonstrate achievement. Typically, the latter includes patient satisfaction data and documentation of activities related to continuing medical education (Wilkinson et al., 2002). They are an opportunity to compare learning accomplishments with learning objectives (Brigden, 1999). Metacognitive features of a portfolio focus on thinking about one's thinking as evident in reflections, self-assessments, and plans.

Specific components that foster metacognitive development are (a) a personal statement of goals for learning that includes awareness of self and others (e.g., institutional expectations); (b) strengths and weaknesses in cognitive, affective, and metacognitive performance, including assessment of learning style; (c) plans for addressing learning needs; (d) self-questions with reflections, plans, and responses compiled during learning experiences; and (e) self-evaluation of performance that includes concordance between self-generated and other sources of data.

Portfolios offer an opportunity to analyze personal and professional growth through continuous review of and reflection on each component. This growth becomes evident in (a) a greater awareness of the progression in personal learning needs and objectives over time, (b) a deeper understanding of one's individual learning style, (c) documentation of a growing list of tailored learning strategies that work ("tips for learning"), and (d) evidence gathered from self and others that supports learning achievements.

Review of Patient's Perspective (RPP)

The learner–patient encounter serves as an opportunity to take another's perspective and compare it to one's own. This includes beliefs, thoughts, and feelings about health and illness. The encounter provides a context for learning from the patient—by viewing the encounter, including one's behaviors, from the patient's point of view. A series of questions for eliciting the patient's perspective can be developed, implemented, and adapted to facilitate such learning. These questions can help the learner achieve specific objectives, such as defining cultural differences between self and the patient or addressing gaps in coordination of care. The series of questions should be integrated into the standard medical history and the referred to as the RPP.

The RPP is an opportunity to elicit the patient's beliefs, concerns, and thoughts about the reason for the encounter (e.g., chief complaint, procedure, and so on). This could include the patient's chief concern (worry about the nature, cause, or impact of the illness or procedure), beliefs about causality and cure (ethnic and religious or psychological developmental—concrete or formal thinking) (Bibace & Walsh, 1980), feelings about self (guilt or shame), and view of the illness or management plan (as constructed with input from others, including family, friends, and other health care professionals). The following sample questions could constitute an RPP:

> What concerns you most about your illness?
>
> What's your understanding of your medical problem? How you developed it? What its course may be like?
>
> Do you have any religious or spiritual concerns about the problem? Do others around you?
>
> Who do you turn to for support or help with your illness?
>
> Who have you talked to (family/friends/other doctors) about it? What have they said?
>
> Do you have any questions? What do you expect (to feel/it to be like)?
>
> Do you know who is in charge of your care and whom to ask questions?

Using the RPP as a foundation, teachers can incorporate perspective taking into the routine of the medical interview. In addition to eliciting the history of present illness (HPI), past medical history (PMH), personal social history (PSH), and review of systems (ROS), students could learn to elicit the RPP. Not only will they be expected to elicit the RPP, they would be expected to incorporate the findings into the oral presentation, problem list, and management plan.

SUMMARY: INTEGRATING METACOGNITIVE SKILL BUILDING INTO THE CURRICULUM

Metacognition is developed within a learning context that fosters self-directed learning and independence. There is evidence in the literature to suggest that learners (particularly medical students) value clinical learning experiences that rely on independence (Lawrence, Lindemann, & Gottlieb, 2000). Programs that are successful in achieving self-directed learning outcomes emphasize the importance of strategic thinking, expose learners to an array of implementation methods (including diaries, practice, role play, and modeling), and provide them with reminders for strategic actions. In the successful programs, there is generally a progression from shared-direction to self-directed learning. There is some evidence that engagement in self-directed learning can lead to achievement of critical capabilities of expertise, such as making independent judgments (Sanson-Fisher, Rolfe, Jones, Ringland, & Agrez, 2002). New strategies, such as reading for (metacognitive) comprehension, developing the learning portfolio, and implementing the RPP, will facilitate self-directed learning during medical school and a lifetime of medical practice.

CHAPTER ELEVEN

A New Curricular Paradigm for Medical Education

INTRODUCTION

In this final chapter, the features of a curriculum that support metacognition and the development of expertise are discussed. Central to the discussion is the notion that the culture, including the values, language, rules, and aims of the medical school and medical education, must support the new paradigm. The culture is reflected in the formal and the hidden curriculum. Both must embrace the experiential world of the learner.

A NEW PARADIGM

The aim of medical education is to develop medical expertise that consists of intuition and metacognition. Both are modes of acting on experience, and the context defines which of the two modes is preferable. Their development is interrelated. Conscious and deliberate analysis of experience (i.e., metacognition) will improve subsequent intuition. Thus, adopting teaching and learning strategies devoted to improving metacognitive capabilities will improve intuition as well. As Hogarth (2001, p. 224) states, "Paradoxically, one result of educating your intuition will be that you allocate more time to directing your deliberate thought processes."

The current curricular paradigm of medical education does not fully support the development of medical expertise or lifelong learning. Neither intuition nor metacognition is systematically fostered or evaluated.

125

Characteristically, the curriculum is defined parochially by the number of hours, days, or weeks that teachers are in proximity of students (i.e., in courses and clerkships). The new paradigm must refocus the centrality of learning within a broader experiential context. Accepting the new paradigm requires renewing the beliefs, assumptions, rules of operation, values, language, and rituals inherent in medical education. It must include learning time no matter what the context and the "hidden" curricula—unwritten goals for students, faculty attitudes toward teaching, and formal and informal communication between students and teachers. The curriculum must also prepare the learner for the "future" classroom—clinical practice.

CULTURE OF MEDICAL EDUCATION

The central values of learning in today's medical school course work and clerkships (i.e., the formal curriculum) revolve around the development of a soon-to-be-outdated knowledge and skill base that can be applied in the present. The language consists primarily of current information and facts, and the rituals of learning emphasize informing, memorizing, and reciting. Although critical for immediate application, these cultural conditions do not prepare the student for future learning and the practice of medicine. Assumptions underlying the current culture are that (a) the focus of teaching and learning should be on mastering *current* knowledge, skills, and attitudes; (b) to learn effectively, students must take good notes, test well, and apply current knowledge and experience to solving clinical problems; and (c) teaching should enhance performance *now* and evaluation should focus on *what was* learned and mastered. In contrast, the new "culture of expertise" in medical education must focus on the future as well as the present and ensure that continuous learning will take place.

There is little evidence in today's paradigm that reflects the fact that the learners in medical school are adults. It is critical to feed the adult learner's hunger for challenging, meaningful learning that will guide future practice (Lanzilotti, 1989). The curriculum therefore must include strategies to address future learning needs and interests as well as the knowledge and skills required to learn (practice) medicine today. These strategies must enable learners to develop *capabilities* (related to both thinking and doing) to manage complexity in medical practice today as well as to continue learning throughout their lives. The development of these capabilities enables the learner to practice medicine now and in the future. As Fraser and Greenhalgh (2001, p. 800) state, "Learning which builds capability takes place when individuals engage with an uncertain and unfamiliar context in a meaningful way."

Students are constantly learning (cognitively, intuitively, and meta-cognitively) from their experiences within the culture in which they are immersed. This includes the formal and the *hidden* curriculum. Students may learn in the formal curriculum that the building blocks of metacognition and intuition are important, but this may be negatively reinforced in the hidden curriculum. For example, the current culture of medical education may not adequately value interpersonal aspects of communication that lead to the development of clinical expertise. Often this culture covertly discourages expression of feelings and reflection (Hafferty & Franks, 1994). It does this by reinforcing only the acquisition of knowledge and technical skills. In a culture dominated by medical language, little attention is paid to language that describes people's thoughts, feelings, and behaviors.

In the current paradigm, students may be getting *mixed messages about what is and is not valuable to learn*. In this regard, Coulihan and Williams (2001) distinguish between the explicit and the tacit values that drive the current culture of medical education. They contend that interpersonal skills that are essential to metacognitive learning, while espoused in parts of the formal curriculum such as introductory courses in clinical medicine, are considered secondary because they are not given status in most cultural areas that count, such as evaluation. These skills, although evident in the words of wisdom espoused by faculty, may not even be reinforced by their preceptors' behaviors.

The tacit values reinforced in the hidden curriculum perpetuate a *social order* that is grounded in the standards and values of technical competence. The current culture fosters specializations and division of labor and is not oriented toward development of a generalized set of thinking skills. As Wear and Castellani (2000, p. 607) state, "Rather than a well-crafted, four year experience where the skills, attitudes, and values relevant to undifferentiated physicians are developed and encouraged, most medical curricula are focused on differentiation and hierarchies of knowledge, on clearly defined spheres of practice, and on controlled distinctions among medical specialties." The specialties that are most closely aligned with the technical aspects of medicine are most highly reinforced by tacit learning.

This hidden curriculum may be most influential in the learning process. That is, medical students may be more likely to adopt behaviors related to what is done rather than what is said. As Coulihan and Williams (2001, p. 600) state, "The explicit curriculum stresses empathy and associated listening and responding skills, the relief of suffering, the importance of trust and fidelity, and a primary focus on the patient's best interest. Tacit learning, on the other hand, stresses objectivity, detachment, wariness, and distrust of emotions, patients, insurance companies, administrators, and the state." Developing metacognition and intuition within such a culture is practically impossible.

The need to establish transparency or alignment of the hidden and formal curricula can be addressed by empowering students to participate in defining learning goals and allowing them to monitor and improve relationships in the learning environment. This should include encouraging them to question the status quo.

Some important strides have already been made in these areas. For example, at one medical school, students in discussion groups gradually take the role of teachers as the cases they discuss become more complex (ten Cate & Smal, 2002). In other medical schools, parts of the culture have already broadened to provide an ideal context for metacognitive development. Students in the very first year are often exposed to a multiplicity of perspectives of health care providers, patients, and resource personnel. The Community Medicine Clerkship at the University of Massachusetts, the Rush Medical School Community Service Initiative, and the University of Toronto Health Illness and Community Program are all examples of learning contexts that can promote metacognitive capability early in medical education (Eckenfels, 1997).

One school is offering more widespread cultural change that addresses the hidden curriculum. The Indiana University School of Medicine has introduced narratives and storytelling to chronicle the transformation of the medical school environment into a "mindful" and "virtuous" place of learning (Suchman, 2004). They are breaking down the traditional barriers between formal and informal (or hidden) curricula by fostering a climate of transparency, equality, and reflection among students and faculty. They have used techniques of interviewing, storytelling, and the open forum to engage learners in the dynamic process of changing the culture of medical education. Early results demonstrate increased feelings of "collegiality of kindred spirits" and "encouragement for learning and personal growth" (Suchman, 2004, p. 502).

THE FORMAL CURRICULUM

Competencies and Objectives

The focus on competencies provides an ideal context for integrating metacognition into the medical school curriculum. Key performance indices from multiple competency areas are beginning to be grouped and organized sequentially to represent developmental milestones in medical school curricula. Metacognitive competencies related to the capabilities defined in chapter 3 can be introduced with cognitive and affective competencies into these curricula to address the full scope of learning in topic areas. The following example shows this.

By the end of the second year, students will be competent in basic communication. They will be able to use basic skills such as open questions to elicit personal social history from people from different cultural backgrounds. They will feel comfortable eliciting sensitive information from patients with different cultural backgrounds. This will include reflecting on and understanding their own feelings and taking the perspectives of others.

The new formal curriculum requires a culture shift from teacher-directed curriculum to shared direction in defining the curriculum. Faculty members must actively and comfortably teach students to develop and implement their own curricula. This will include helping students (a) define and prioritize their goals, (b) anticipate and assess their specific needs in relation to the goals, (c) organize (and reorganize) their experiences to meet their unique needs, (d) define their own and recognize differences in others' perspectives, and (e) continuously monitor their knowledge base, problem solving, and interactions with others. These are the capabilities of metacognition.

Several studies provide empirical evidence that self-assessment, self-monitoring, planning, and reflection can be developed with teachers' help within a structured curriculum and that learners can become better and more autonomous thinkers as a result (Hernstein, Nickerson, Sanchez, & Swets, 1986; Perkins & Grotzer, 1997; Shain, 1992; Williams et al., 1996; Zimmerman, 1995). Research suggests that developing the metacognitive skills to learn from experience, particularly those that are used for monitoring understanding and assessing comprehension, can be developed in college and beyond (Koriat & Goldsmith, 1996; Perfect & Schwartz, 2002). Research also suggests that medical school faculty can play an important role in facilitating preclinical students' acquisition of metacognitive capabilities that will improve outcomes of learning throughout a lifetime (Palincsar & Brown, 1984).

In the new curriculum, faculty must use appropriate teaching methods to help learners develop metacognitive competencies. For example, previewing how one "briefly" plans the patient interview in the seconds before one walks into the exam room is an important teaching strategy that is often overlooked. Unless these changes are formally adopted at the curricular level, with guidance from the clerkship director, the chances of the preceptor fostering and properly evaluating the *expert behavior* of students in the clinical learning setting will be *hit or miss*. In fact, the current paradigm with its emphasis on content is likely to reinforce less than expert behavior, such as recall of factual knowledge, and dismiss attempts to plan and reflect on experience.

The context for learning in the new paradigm is being defined by forces beyond the control of medical school curriculum developers. It is increasingly evident that clinical teachers are rarely available to take advantage of the "teachable moment" with their learners. Increased responsibilities for patient care and practice management take precedence for the physician-teacher. Often, when faculty members do have time, they teach at the cognitive level—providing information or directions for how to do something—rather than teach learners how to think about their thinking. More than occasionally, learners become *leaners* and rely on teachers for basic help. Rarely do medical teachers share their opinion or their views about what they or their patients are thinking or probe the learner's thoughts about his or her thinking.

In the clinical years, students are placed in a variety of "educational" situations in which they are expected to learn independently of the teacher. Often these situations include learning from others—patients, peers, and team members. Even if the learning involves others, it always includes learning from self. Largely, medical students are their own curriculum developers. They must be prepared to predict and anticipate the time and place in which important learning could occur, and they must be formally equipped to ensure the occurrence of such learning.

Teachers can no longer be expected to provide only information and direction. They are models who become the focus of learner observation, self-questioning, and reflection. In addition, they serve as guides to help learners navigate through readily available information and as "facilitators of thinking and acting." Studies have shown that teaching metacognitive strategies can better help learners transfer learning to new situations, which is the ultimate test of the new curriculum (Brown, Palincsar, & Armbruster, 1984).

The redefinition of roles of teacher and learner and the expansion of the goals, content, time frame, and context of medical education all point to the critical role the learner must play in the learning process. In the new paradigm, learners are not taught to become health care providers during medical school and residency. Instead, they begin to develop and, most important, practice thinking skills *at the beginning of medical school* that will enable them to learn, care for patients, and teach others *throughout their lifetimes.* They seek out and are provided with opportunities to gain self-awareness from experience. The value of developing personal awareness to "one's professional role as a healer has been noted by others" (Longhurst, 1988, p. 121).

It is with great insight that the forefathers of medicine chose the term "practice" to describe their patient care activities. The beginning learner develops and refines capabilities of intuition and metacognition early in training and assumes more responsibility for learning from experience and teaching others while caring for patients. The benefits of experience to learning, practice, and teaching are mutual and intertwined.

Knowledge is critical to the new curriculum. In addition to gaining knowledge, medical students need to develop metaknowledge—"knowledge involving higher-order evaluation of lower-order information" (Lehrer, 1990, p. 254). This includes recognizing what they know and don't know, how they best learn what they need, how to develop and implement a plan to obtain what they need, and the ability to monitor their success in getting there. Assumptions underlying the "new" culture are that (a) learners must be prepared to master new competencies *throughout their lives;* (b) to learn throughout their lives, students need to *be aware of their learning and to practice effective learning strategies;* and (c) teaching and evaluation must focus on learning in the *future.*

The new learning context in medical education focuses on the experiential world of the learner. In this new context, there must be a "shift from a regulation of the student learning process by teachers and school to self-regulation of learning" (ten Cate et al., 2004, p. 221). Ultimately, the new context for learning is the experience of learning itself. In this context, the learner continuously relies on personal awareness of his or her behavior, beliefs, strengths, and weaknesses in relation to surrounding activities (Scardamalia & Bereiter, 1985; Sternberg, 1985). During the first year of medical school, faculty members can promote an awareness of the concepts of metacognition and intuition, introduce specific strategies to enhance capabilities related to both, and structure the learning environment to promote growth in experiential thinking (Hartman & Sternberg, 1993; Hogarth, 2001).

Focus on Experience

The key to developing medical expertise is to enable learners to recognize when and how to activate the learning process. Employing intuition involves the capability to both recognize patterns and accurately match key features to experience gained through previous conceptual (text) or active learning. Klein (1998, p. 42) suggests, "The part of intuition that involves pattern matching and recognition of familiar and typical cases can be trained." The accuracy of intuition and metacognition depends on the accuracy of observation and ability to store for recall. Teaching strategies can be adopted to increase the validity and reliability of observation and the *quality of experience.* Hogarth (2001, p. 223) says that "to educate intuition it is necessary to improve the ability to learn accurately from experience." Finally, increasing the quantity and breadth of experience—the raw material for learning—will ultimately enhance the experience base from which to draw. In the new culture of teaching and learning, the following is true: (a) learners help identify situations for learning; (b) learning from experience includes learning from self as well as others; (c) eliciting, analyzing, and accepting feedback from others is critical to learning; and (d) learning is every day for the rest of your life.

Evaluation

There is evidence that metacognition is related to achievement. The findings show that high achievers possess greater metacognitive capability than low-achieving learners (Sternberg, 1985). This would suggest that medical students as a group have greater potential to become metacognitive and ultimately intuitive thinkers. It also suggests that evaluating metacognitive development throughout medical school provides critical data on performance potential of learners.

New strategies are required to evaluate metacognitive and intuitive performance and can be integrated into current evaluation designs that measure cognitive and affective outcomes. Within an integrated framework, it is expected that students will begin to obtain metacognitive knowledge and skills along with cognitive and affective capability early in medical school and continue to enhance their expertise throughout their professional careers. Capabilities in each of these areas should be measured using specifically designed evaluation strategies.

Measuring metacognition will involve examining expected outcomes associated with each capability related to both regulatory strategies and strategic knowledge. Ideally, these evaluation strategies will be interwoven with current strategies. For instance, the capability to take the patient's perspective can be evaluated by preceptors and attendings through the oral presentation. Students and residents could be expected to present the RPP along with the history of present illness, past medical history, and review of systems. Formative feedback from teachers that focuses on history-taking and interviewing skills will include assessment of observed behavior and presentation skills related to the RPP. Final evaluation checklists completed by faculty and preceptors will include the RPP along with other prominent features of the patient history.

The capability to reflect and monitor behavior can be evaluated through formal mechanisms, such as the experiential narrative. Students could be required to submit narratives at the end of their mandatory introductory clinical medicine course to be judged on the quality of reflection and personal awareness. Other outcomes related to metacognitive capabilities, such as reading comprehension strategies, will be measured through more traditional means, such as written exams. An effective evaluation process in the new paradigm will include strategies for measuring cognitive, affective, and metacognitive capabilities throughout the continuum, including continuing medical education.

Evaluating the development of expertise also will include evaluation of intuition or rapid cognition. This will demand a different testing technique as well as different testing conditions. A creative solution has been posed by Schmidt, Norman, and Boshuizen (1990, p. 619), who have called for "staged testing." Under these conditions, students would initially "be challenged with a large variety of presenting situations, each with minimal information, under time constraints, and asked to arrive at a solution as quickly as possible" (p. 620). The result would provide a measure of the extent to which students have attained expertise in the "rapid, non-analytic" dimension that characterizes intuition (p. 619). In this staged approach, students could be given extra time to apply analytic and even metacognitive skills to the problems they did not finish or were not able to answer correctly. They could assess their knowledge with respect to the problem, reflect on the assumptions they made (CBRs), and offer and test alternative solutions. Both formatively and summatively, students could be evaluated and receive feedback on the application of their thinking skills as well as the proposed solutions they offer. One would expect that over the course of learning throughout the continuum, many more problems would be solved rapidly as experience and expertise grow.

SUMMARY

Constructing and implementing the new paradigm for medical education that aims to develop medical expertise demands restructuring of the basic principles that have driven medical education for so long. First and foremost is a new appreciation for the value of learning from experience. However, learning from experience is not independent learning. Preparing learners to think about how they think, consider what they know (and don't know), discover how they feel, and compare their experiences demands significant *up-front* curriculum time and faculty effort. In essence, teachers can promote the development of these capabilities by adopting teaching strategies that encourage learners to actively engage in experiential learning and adopt rules of thinking that will facilitate the development of a lifelong personalized curriculum. The personalized curriculum that is the hallmark of the new paradigm begins in the first year of medical school with the establishment of an infrastructure for thinking that will impact learning, practice, and teaching. New evaluation strategies must focus on the achievement of metacognitive as well as cognitive benchmarks and capabilities.

References

Abernathy, C. M., & Hamm, R. M. (1995). *Surgical intuition: What it is and how to get it.* Philadelphia: Hanley & Belfus.

Abernathy, C. M., & Harken, A. H. (Eds.). (1991). *Surgical secrets* (2nd ed.). Philadelphia: Hanley & Belfus.

Accreditation Council for Graduate Medical Education. (2005). *Outcomes project.* Retrieved September 5, 2005, 2005, from http://www.acgme.org/outcome

Ainoda, N., Onishi, H., & Yasuda, Y. (2005). Definitions and goals of "self-directed learning" in contemporary medical education literature. *Annals of the Academy of Medicine, Singapore, 34*(8), 515–520.

Airey, N., Marriott, J., & Rodd, J. (2001). Learning styles of psychiatrists and other specialists. *Psychiatric Bulletin, 25,* 306–309.

Ambady, N., & Gray, H. M. (2002). On being sad and mistaken: Mood effects on the accuracy of thin-slice judgments. *Journal of Personality and Social Psychology, 83*(4), 947–961.

Ambady, N., LaPlante, D., Nguyen, T., Rosenthal, R., Chaumeton, N., & Levinson, W. (2002). Surgeons' tone of voice: A clue to malpractice history. *Surgery, 132*(1), 5–9.

Ambady, N., & Rosenthal, R. (1992). Thin slices of behavior as predictors of interpersonal consequences: A meta-analysis. *Psychological Bulletin, 2,* 256–274.

Ambady, N., & Rosenthal, R. (1993). Half a minute: Predicting teacher evaluations from thin slices of nonverbal behavior and physical attractiveness. *Journal of Personality and Social Psychology, 64*(3), 431–441.

Antonelli, M. A. S. (1997). Accuracy of second-year medical students' self-assessment of clinical skills. *Academic Medicine, 72*(Suppl. 10), S63–S65.

Argyris, C. (1989). *Reasoning, learning and action.* San Francisco: Jossey-Bass.

Ayres, I. (2002). *Pervasive prejudice? Unconventional evidence of race and gender discrimination.* Chicago: University of Chicago Press.

Baker, W. D. (1989). *Reading skills: Improving speed and comprehension* (3rd ed.). Englewood Cliffs, NJ: Prentice Hall.

Bargh, J. A., Chen, M., & Burrows, L. (1996). Automaticity of social behavior: Direct effects of trait construct and stereotype activation on action. *Journal of Personality and Social Psychology, 71*(2), 230–244.

Barnsley, L., Lyon, P. M., Ralston, S. J., Hibbert, E. J., Cunningham, F. C., & Field, M. J. (2004). Clinical skills in junior medical officers: A comparison of self-reported confidence and observed competence. *Medical Education, 38,* 358–367.

Bar-On, R. (2000). Emotional and social intelligence: Insights from the Emotional Quotient Inventory. In R. Bar-On & J. D. A. Parker (Eds.), *The handbook of emotional intelligence* (pp. 363–388). San Francisco: Jossey-Bass.

Baron, R. M., & Boudreau, L. A. (1987). An ecological perspective on integrating personality and social psychology. *Journal of Personality and Social Psychology, 53*(6), 1222–1228.

Bechara, A., Damasio, H., Tranel, D., & Damasio, A. (1997, February 28). Deciding advantageously before knowing the advantageous strategy. *Science, 275,* 1293–1295.

Bibace, R., & Walsh, M. E. (1980). Development of children's concepts of illness. *Pediatrics, 66*(6), 912–917.

Billings, J. (1887). Methods of research in medical literature. *Transactions of the Association of American Physicians, 2,* 57–67.

Blumberg, P., & Michael, J. A. (1992). Development of self-directed learning behaviors in partially teacher-directed problem-based learning curriculum. *Teaching and Learning in Medicine, 4*(1), 3–8.

Boenink, A. D., Oderwald, A. K., De Jong, P., Van Tilburg, W., & Smal, L. A. (2004). Assessing student reflection in medical practice. The development of an observer-rated instrument: Reliability, validity, and initial experience. *Medical Education, 38,* 368–377.

Bordage, G., & Lemieux, M. (1990). Which medical textbook to read? Emphasizing semantic structures. *Academic Medicine, 65*(Suppl.), 23S–24S.

Borkan, J., Reis, S., & Medalie, J. (2001). Narratives in family medicine: Tales of transformation, points of breakthrough for family physicians. *Families, Systems and Health, 19*(2), 121–131.

Brenner, L., Koehler, D., Liberman, V., & Tversky, A. (1996). Overconfidence in probability and frequency judgments: A critical examination. *Organizational Behavior and Human Decision Processes, 65,* 212–219.

Brigden, D. (1999, July 7). Constructing a learning portfolio. *British Medical Journal, 319,* 2.

Britton, B. K., Stimson, M., Stennett, B., & Gulgoz, S. (1998). Learning from instructional text: Test of an individual difference model. *Journal of Educational Psychology, 90,* 476–491.

Brookfield, S. (1981). Independent adult learning. *Studies in Adult Education, 13*(1), 15–27.

Brookfield, S. (1993). Self-directed learning, political clarity, and the critical practice of adult education. *Adult Education Quarterly, 43*(4), 227–242.

Brookfield, S. D. (1995). *Becoming a critically reflective teacher.* San Francisco: Jossey-Bass.

Brown, A. L. (1978). Knowing when, where and how to remember: A problem for metacognition. In R. Glaser (Ed.), *Advances in instructional psychology* (Vol. 1, pp. 77–165). Hillsdale NJ: Erlbaum.

Brown, A. L., & Campione, J. C. (1977). Training strategic study time apportionment in educatable retarded children. *Intelligence, 1,* 94–107.

Brown, A. L., Palincsar, A. S., & Armbruster, B. B. (1984). Instructing comprehension fostering activities in interactive learning situations. In H. Mandl, N. L. Stein, & T. Trabasso (Eds.), *Learning and comprehension of text* (pp. 255–290). Hillsdale, NJ: Erlbaum.

Butler, D. L., & Winne, P. H. (1995). Feedback and self-regulated learning: A theoretical synthesis. *Review of Educational Research, 65,* 245–281.

Calleigh, A. S. (Ed.) (2000). Professionalism [Special issue]. *Academic Medicine, 75*(6).

Candy, P. C. (1991). *Self direction for lifelong learning: A comprehensive guide to theory and practice.* San Francisco: Jossey-Bass.

Carraccio, C., & Englander, R. (2004). Evaluating competence using a portfolio: A literature review and web-based application to the ACGME competencies. *Teaching and Learning in Medicine, 16*(4), 381–387.

Chauhan, S. P., Magann, E. F., McAninch, C. B., Gherman, R. B., & Morrison, J. C. (2003). Application of learning theory to obstetric maloccurrence. *Journal of Maternal Fetal and Neonatal Medicine, 13*(3), 203–207.

Claridge, L. (2003, September 14). Medicine man: Tracy Kidder profiles Dr. Paul Farmer, a modern-day Robin Hood hoping to wipe out infectious disease. *Boston Globe,* p. D8.

Coulihan, J., & Williams, P. C. (2001, June). Vanquishing virtue: The impact of medical education. *Academic Medicine, 76,* 598–605.

Crandall, B., & Getchell-Reiter, K. (1993). Critical decision method: A technique for eliciting concrete assessment indicators from the "intuition" of NICU nurses. *Advances in Nursing Science, 16*(1), 42–51.

Croskerry, P. (2003). The importance of cognitive errors in diagnosis and strategies to minimize them. *Academic Medicine, 78*(8), 775–780.

Curry, L. (1999). Cognitive and learning styles in medical education. *Academic Medicine, 74*(4), 409–413.

Davidson, J. E., Deuser, R., & Sternberg, R. J. (1994). The role of metacognition in problem solving. In J. Metcalfe & A. P. Shimamura (Eds.), *Metacognition: Knowing about knowing* (pp. 207–226). Cambridge, MA: MIT Press.

Davies, S. M., Rutledge, C. M., & Davies, T. C. (1995). Students' learning styles do affect performance [Letter to the editor]. *Academic Medicine, 70*(8), 659–660.

Davis, M. (1980). A multidimensional approach to individual differences in empathy. *Catalog of Selected Documents in Psychology, 10, 85.*

Davis, M. (1983). Measuring individual differences in empathy: Evidence for a multidimensional approach. *Journal of Personality and Social Psychology, 44, 113–126.*

Denes-Raj, V., & Epstein, S. (1994). Conflict between intuitive and rational processing: When people behave against their better judgment. *Journal of Personality and Social Psychology, 66*(5), 819–829.

Deshler, D. D., & Schumaker, J. B. (1988). An instructional model for teaching students how to learn. In J. L. Graden, J. E. Zins & M. J. Curtis (Eds.), *Alternative educational delivery systems: Enhancing instructional options for all students* (pp. 391–411). National Association of School Psychologists.

Dictionary. (2005). Microsoft Word. Retrieved August 25, 2005.

Dreyfus, H. L., & Dreyfus, S. E. (1986). *Mind over machine.* New York: Free Press.

Duffy, F. D., Gordon, G. H., Whelan, G., Cole-Kelly, K., & Frankel, R. (2004). Assessing competence in communication and interpersonal skills: The Kalamazoo II report. *Academic Medicine, 79*(6), 495–507.

Dunn, R., & Dunn, K. (1993). *Teaching secondary students through their individual learning styles.* Boston: Allyn and Bacon.

Eckenfels, E. J. (1997). Contemporary medical students' quest for self-fulfillment through community service. *Academic Medicine, 72*(12), 1043–1050.

Ende, J. (1983). Feedback in clinical medical education. *Journal of the American Medical Association, 250, 777–781.*

Feltovich, P. J., & Barrows, H. S. (1984). Issues of generality in medical problem-solving. In H. G. Schmidt & M. L. deVolder (Eds.), *Tutorials in problem-based learning: A new direction in teaching the health professions* (pp. 128–142). Assen: Van Gorcum.

Fernandez-Duque, D., Baird, J. A., & Posner, M. I. (2000). Executive attention and metacognitive regulation. *Consciousness and Cognition, 9, 288–307.*

Fitzgerald, J. T., White, C. B., and Gruppen, L. D. (2003). A longitudinal study of self-assessment accuracy. *Medical Education, 37, 645–649.*

Flavell, J. H. (1976). Metacognitive aspects of problem solving. In L. B. Resnick (Ed.), *The nature of intelligence* (pp. 231–235). Hillsdale, NJ: Erlbaum.

Flavell, J. H. (1979). Metacognition and cognitive monitoring: A new area of cognitive-developmental inquiry. *American Psychologist, 34, 906–911.*

Flavell, J. H., Miller, P. H., & Miller, S. A. (1985). *Cognitive development* (4th ed.). Englewood Cliffs, NJ: Prentice Hall.

Forgas, J. P. (1998). On being happy and mistaken: Mood effects on the fundamental attribution error. *Journal of Personality and Social Psychology, 75, 318–331.*

Fowler, J. (1978). Mapping faith's structures: A developmental overview. In J. Fowler, S. Keen, & J. Berryman (Eds.), *Life-maps: The human journey of human faith* (pp. 94–96). Needham Heights, MA: Humanities Press.

Fraser, S. W., & Greenhalgh, T. (2001, October 6). Coping with complexity: Educating for capability. *British Medical Journal, 323, 799–803.*

Gardner, H. (1983). *Frames of mind: The theory of multiple intelligences*. New York: Basic Books.

Gladwell, M. (2005). *Blink*. New York: Little, Brown.

Goldberger, P. (2002). Dept. of delay: A Gehry for Los Los Angeles. *New Yorker, 78*(3), 29.

Goldman, L., Cook, E. F., Johnson, P. A., Brand, D. A., Rouan, G. W., & Lee, T. H. (1996). Prediction of the need for intensive care in patients who come to emergency departments with acute chest pain. *New England Journal of Medicine, 334*(23), 1498–1504.

Goleman, D. (1995). *Emotional intelligence: Why it can matter*. New York: Bantam.

Gordon, M. J. (1991). A review of the validity and accuracy of self-assessments in health professions training. *Academic Medicine, 66*, 762–769.

Gordon, M. J. (1992). Self-assessment programs and their implications for health professions training. *Academic Medicine, 67*, 672–679.

Graber, M. (2003). Metacognitive training to reduce diagnostic errors: Ready for prime time? *Academic Medicine, 78*(8), 781.

Greenhalgh, T. (2002, May). Intuition and evidence—Uneasy bedfellows? *British Journal of General Practice, 52*(478), 394–400.

Greenwald, A., McGhee, D., & Schwartz, J. (1998). Measuring individual difference in implicit cognition: The Implicit Association Test. *Journal of Personality and Social Psychology, 74*(6), 1464–1480.

Greer, M. (2005). When intuition misfires. *APA Monitor, 36*(3), 58–60.

Gruppen, L. D., Garcia, J., Grum, C. M., Fitzgerald, J. T., White, C. A., Dicken, L., Sisson, J. C., & Zweifler, A. (1997). Medical students' self-assessment accuracy in communication skills. *Academic Medicine, 72*(Suppl. 10), S57–S59.

Gunzburger, L. (1980). Characteristics identified upon entrance to medical school associated with future participation in professional education (Doctoral dissertation, University of Chicago, 1980). *Dissertation Abstracts International, 41*, 2572A.

Hafferty, F. W. & Franks, R. (1994). The hidden curriculum, ethics teaching, and the structure of medical education. *Academic Medicine, 69*(11), 861–871.

Hartman, H. J. (Ed.). (2001). *Metacognition in learning and instruction: Theory, research, and practice*. Dordrecht: Kluwer Academic Publishers.

Hartman, H. J., & Sternberg, R. (1993). A broad BACEIS for improving thinking. *Instructional Science, 21*, 401–425.

Harvey, B. J., Rothman, A. I., & Frecker, R. C. (2003). Effect of an undergraduate medical curriculum on students' self-directed learning. *Academic Medicine, 78*(12), 1259–1265.

Hernstein, R. J., Nickerson, R. S., Sanchez, M., & Swets, J. A. (1986). Teaching thinking skills. *American Psychologist, 41*, 1279–1289.

Hogarth, R. (2001). *Educating intuition*. Chicago: University of Chicago Press.

Horiszny, J. A. (2001). Teaching cardiac auscultation using simulated heart sounds and small-group discussion. *Family Medicine, 33*(1), 39–44.

Israel, S. E., Block, C. C., Bauserman, K. L., & Kinnucan-Welsch (Eds.). (2005). *Metacognition in literacy learning: Theory, assessment, instruction, and professional development*. Mahwah, NJ: Erlbaum.

Judge, T. A., & Cable, D. M. (2004). The effect of physical height on workplace success and income: Preliminary test of a theoretical model. *Journal of Applied Psychology, 89*(3), 428–441.

Kidder, T. (2003). *Mountains beyond mountains: The quest of Paul Farmer, a man who would cure the world*. New York: Random House.

King, A. (1991). Effects of training in strategic questions on children's problem solving performance. *Journal of Educational Psychology, 83*, 307–317.

Kitchener, K. S. (1986). The reflective judgment model: Characteristics, evidence, and measurement. In R. A. Mines & K. S. Kitchener (Eds.), *Adult cognitive development: Methods and models* (pp. 76–91). New York: Praeger.

Kitchener, K. S., & Brenner, H. (1990). Wisdom and reflective judgment: Knowing in the face of uncertainty. In R. Sternberg (Ed.), *Wisdom: Its nature, origins and development* (pp. 212–229). Cambridge: Cambridge University Press.

Kittridge, R. W., & Heywood, C. A. (2000). Metacognition and awareness. *Consciousness and Cognition, 9*, 308–312.

Klein, G. (1998). *Sources of power.* Cambridge, MA: MIT Press.

Kleinman, A. (1988). *The illness narratives: Suffering, healing and the human condition.* New York: Basic Books.

Kluwe, R. H. (1982). Cognitive knowledge and executive control: Metacognition. In D. R. Griffin (Ed.), *Animal mind—Human mind* (pp. 201–224). New York: Springer-Verlag.

Kolb, D. (1984). *Experimental learning: Experience as a source of learning and development.* Englewood Cliffs, NJ: Prentice Hall.

Koriat, A., & Goldsmith, M. (1996). Monitoring and control processes in the strategic regulation of memory accuracy. *Psychological Review, 103*, 490–517.

Kowalkzyk, L. (2005, August 31). U.S. study finds rise in state's uninsured. *Boston Globe.*

Kruger, J., & Dunning, D. (1999). Unskilled and unaware of it: How difficulties in recognizing one's own incompetence lead to inflated self-assessments. *Journal of Personality and Social Psychology, 77*(6), 1121–1134.

Kunzmann, U., & Baltes, P. B. (2003). Beyond the traditional scope of intelligence: Wisdom in action. In R. J. Sternberg, J. Lautrey, & T. I. Lubart (Eds.), *Models of intelligence: International perspectives* (1st ed., pp. 329–343). Washington, DC: American Psychological Association.

Lanzilotti, S. (1989). Curiosity. In R. D. Fox, P. E. Mazmanian, & R. W. Putnam (Eds.), *Changing and learning in the lives of physicians* (pp. 29–43). New York: Praeger.

Lave, J., & Wenger, E. (1990). *Situated learning: Legitimate peripheral participation.* Cambridge: Cambridge University Press.

Lawrence, S. L., Lindemann, J. C., & Gottlieb, M. (2000). What students value: Learning outcomes in a required third year ambulatory primary care clerkship. *Medical Education, 34*, 292–298.

Lazare, A. (2004). *On apology.* New York: Oxford University Press.

Lazare, A., Putnam, S., & Lipkin, M. (1995). Three functions of the medical interview. In M. Lipkin, S. Putnam, & A. Lazare (Eds.), *The medical interview* (pp. 3–20). New York: Springer-Verlag.

Lehrer, K. (1990). *Metamind.* Oxford: Clarendon Press.

Levinson, W. W., Roter, D. L., Mullooly, J. P., Dull, V. T., & Frankel, R. M. (1997). Physician-patient communication: The relationship with malpractice claims among primary care physicians and surgeons. *Journal of the American Medical Association, 277*, 553–559.

Lewicki, P., Hill, T., & Bizot, E. (1988). Acquisition of procedural knowledge about a pattern of stimuli that cannot be articulated. *Cognitive Psychology, 20*, 24–37.

Lewicki, P., Hill, T., & Czyzewska, M. (1992). Nonconscious acquisition of information. *The American Psychologist, 47*, 796–801.

Linn, B. S., Arostegui, M., & Zeppa, R. (1975). Performance rating scale for peer and self-assessment. *British Journal of Medical Education, 9*, 98.

Longhurst, M. (1988, July 15). Physician self-awareness: The neglected insight. *Canadian Medical Association Journal, 139*, 121–124.

Losh, D. P., Mauksch, L. B., Arnold, R. W., Maresca, T. M., Storck, M. G., Maestas, R. R., & Goldstein, E. (2005). Teaching inpatient communication skills to medical students: An innovative strategy. *Academic Medicine, 80*(2), 118–124.

Maki, R. H., & Berry, S. L. (1984). Metacomprehension of text material. *Journal of Experimental Psychology, 10,* 663–679.

Maki, R. H., & McGuire, M. J. (2002). Metacognition for text: Implications for education. In T. J. Perfect & B. L. Schwartz (Eds.), *Applied metacognition* (pp. 39–67): Cambridge: Cambridge University Press.

Markakis, K. M., Beckman, H. B., Suchman, A. L., & Frankel, R. M. (2000). The path to professionalism: Cultivating humanistic values and attitudes in residency training. *Academic Medicine, 75*(2), 141–150.

Martin, I. G., Stark, P., & Jolly, B. (2000). Benefiting from clinical experience: The influence of learning style and clinical experience on performance in an undergraduate objective structured clinical examination. *Medical Education, 34,* 530–534.

Mast, T. J., & Davis, D. (1994). Concepts of competence. In D. Davis & R. D. Fox (Eds.), *The physician as learner: Linking research to practice* (pp. 139–156). Chicago: American Medical Association.

Matthews, G., Zeidner, M., & Roberts, R. D. (2002). *Emotional intelligence.* Cambridge, MA: MIT Press.

McCune, S. K., Guglielmino, L. M., & Garcia, G. (1990). Adult self-direction in learning: A preliminary meta-analytic investigation of research using the Self-Directed Learning Readiness Scale. In H. L. Associates (Ed.), *Advances in self-directed learning research* (pp. 145–156). Norman: Oklahoma Research Center for Continuing Professional and Higher Education, University of Oklahoma.

McNeil, D. E., Sandberg, D. A., & Binder, R. L. (1998). The relationship between confidence and accuracy in clinical assessment of psychiatric patient's potential for violence. *Law and Human Behavior,* 655–669.

Metcalfe, J. (1998). Cognitive optimism: Self-deception of memory-based processing heuristics? *Personality and Social Psychology Review, 2,* 100–110.

Miflin, B. M., Campbell, C. B., & Price, D. A. (1999). A lesson from the introduction of a problem-based, graduate entry course: The effects of different views on self-direction. *Medical Education, 33,* 801–807.

Miflin, B. M., Campbell, C. B., & Price, D. A. (2000). A conceptual framework to guide the development of self-directed, lifelong learning in problem-based medical curricula. *Medical Education, 34,* 299–306.

Mitchell, R., & Liu, P. L. (1995). A study of resident learning behavior. *Teaching and Learning in Medicine, 7*(4), 233–240.

Most, D. (2003). The silent treatment. *Boston Magazine,* pp. 105+.

Myers, D. G. (2002). *Intuition.* New Haven, CT: Yale University Press.

Nickerson, R. S., Baddeley, A., & Freeman, B. (1987). Are people's estimates of what other people know influenced by what they themselves know? *Acta Psychologica, 64,* 245–259.

Norman, G. R., Muzzin, C. J., Somers, S., & Rosenthal, D. (1992). Visual perception in medical practice. In H. G. Schmidt, Z. Nooman, & E. Ezzad (Eds.), *Innovation in medical education: An evaluation of its present status* (pp. 204–217). New York: Springer-Verlag.

Novack, D. H., Suchman, A. L., Clark, W., Epstein, R. M., Najberg, E., & Kaplan, C. (1997). Calibrating the physician. *Journal of the American Medical Association, 278*(6), 502–508.

Open University. (1992). *A portfolio approach for personal and career development.* Milton Keynes: Author.

Osler, S. W. (1897). Influence of Louis on American medicine. *Johns Hopkins Hospital Bulletin, 8,* 161.

Palincsar, A., & Brown, A. (1984). Reciprocal teaching of comprehension fostering and monitoring activities. *Cognition and Instruction, 1*(2), 117–175.

Pellegrino, E. D. (2002). Professionalism, profession and the virtues of the good physician. *Mount Sinai Journal of Medicine, 69*(6), 378–384.

Perfect, T. J., & Schwartz, B. L. (Eds.). (2002). *Applied metacognition.* Cambridge: Cambridge University Press.

Perkins, D. N., & Grotzer, T. A. (1997). Teaching intelligence. *American Psychologist, 52*(10), 1125–1133.

Piaget, J. (1972). *The psychology of intelligence.* Totowa, NJ: Littlefield, Adams.

Pressley, M. (2002). Metacognition and self-regulated comprehension. In A. E. Farstrup & S. J. Samuels (Eds.), *What research has to say about reading instruction* (3rd ed., pp. 291–309). Newark, NJ: International Reading Association.

Pressley, M., Goodchild, F., Fleet, J., Zajchowski, R., & Evans, E. D. (1989). The challenges of classroom strategy instruction. *Elementary School Journal, 89,* 301–342.

Pringle, M., Bradley, C. P., Carmichael, C. M., Wallis, H., & Moore, A. (1995). *Significant event auditing: A study of the feasibility and potential of case-based auditing in primary care.* London: RCGP.

Project Professionalism. (1995). *Professionalism in medicine: Issues and opportunities in the educational environment.* Philadelphia: American Board of Internal Medicine.

Quirk, M. E. (1994). *How to learn and teach in medical school: A learner-centered approach.* Springfield, IL: Charles C. Thomas.

Reeves, W. W. (1996). *Cognition and complexity: The cognitive science of managing complexity.* Lanham, MD: Scarecrow Press.

Resnick, R. A. (2004). Visual sensing without seeing. *Psychological Science, 15*(1), 27–32.

Reynolds, M. M. (1986). The self-directedness and motivational orientations of adult part-time students at a community college (Doctoral dissertation, Syracuse University, 1984). *Dissertation Abstracts International, 46,* 571A.

Robinson, A. (1993). *What smart students know.* New York: Crown.

Ross, L., Greene, D., & House, P. (1977). The " false consensus effect": An egocentric bias in social perception and attributional processes. *Journal of Experimental Social Psychology, 13,* 279–301.

Sanson-Fisher, R. W., Rolfe, I. E., Jones, P., Ringland, C., & Agrez, M. (2002). Trialling a new way to learn clinical skills: Systematic clinical appraisal and learning. *Medical Education, 36,* 1028–1034.

Savitsky, K., & Gilovich, T. (2003). The illusion of transparency and the alleviation of speech anxiety. *Journal of Experimental Social Psychology, 39*(6), 618–625.

Scardamalia, M. (2002). Collective cognitive responsibility for the advancement of knowledge. In B. Smith (Ed.), *Liberal education in a knowledge society* (pp. 1–14). Chicago: Open Court.

Scardamalia, M., & Bereiter, C. (1985). Fostering the development of self-regulation in children's knowledge processing. In S. F. Chipman, J. W. Segal, & R. Glaser (Eds.), *Thinking and learning skills, Vol 2: Research and open questions* (pp. 563–577). Hillsdale, NJ: Erlbaum.

Schmidt, H. G. (2000). Assumptions underlying self-directed learning may be false. *Medical Education, 34,* 243–245.

Schmidt, H. G., Norman, G. R., & Boshuizen, H. P. A. (1990). A cognitive perspective on medical expertise: Theory and implications. *Academic Medicine, 65*(10), 611–621.

Schön, D. A. (1987). *Educating the reflective practitioner: Toward a new design for teaching and learning in the professions.* San Francisco: Jossey-Bass.

Schooler, J. W., & Engstler-Schooler, T. Y. (1990). Verbal overshadowing of visual memories: Some things are better left unsaid. *Cognitive Psychology, 22,* 36–71.

Sclabassi, S. E., & Woelfel, S. K. (1984). Development of self-assessment skills in medical students. *Medical Education, 84,* 226–231.

Selman. R. L. (1971). The relation of role taking to the development of moral judgment in children. *Child Development, 42,* 79–91.

Shain, D. (1992). *Study skills and test taking strategies for medical students.* New York: Springer-Verlag.

Shields, S. (2005). *Personal narrative.* Unpublished manuscript.

Shirlley, D. A., & Langan-Fox, J. (1996). Intuition: A review of the literature. *Psychological Reports, 79,* 563–584.

Shokar, G. S., Shokar, N. K., Romero, C. M., & Bulik, R. J. (2002). Self-directed learning: Looking at outcomes with medical students. *Family Medicine, 34*(3), 197–200.

Shulman, K. A., Berlin, J. A., Harless, W., Kerner, J. F., Systrunk, S., Gersh, B. J., Dube, R., Talegahni, C. K., Burke, J. E., Williams, S., Eisenberg, J. M., & Escarce, J. J. (1999). The effect of race and sex on physicians' recommendations for cardiac catheterization. *New England Journal of Medicine, 340*(8), 618–626.

Simon, H. A. (1992). What is an "explanation" of behavior. *Psychological Science, 3,* 150–161.

Simpson, M. L., & Nist, S. L. (2002). Encouraging active reading at the college level. In C. Collins Block & M. Pressley (Eds.), *Comprehension instruction* (pp. 365–379). New York: Guilford.

Smith, L. H. (1985). Medical education for the 21st century. *Journal of Medical Education, 60,* 106–112.

Son, L. K., & Schwartz, B. L. (2002). Relation between metacognitive monitoring and control. In T. J. Perfect & B. L. Schwartz (Eds.), *Applied metacognition* (pp. 15–38). Cambridge: Cambridge University Press.

Starr, S., Ferguson, W. J., Haley, H.-L., & Quirk, M. (2003). Community preceptors' views of their identities as teachers. *Academic Medicine, 78*(8), 820–825.

Sternberg, R. (1985). *Beyond IQ.* Cambridge: Cambridge University Press.

Sternberg, R. (1997a). The concept of intelligence and its role in lifelong learning and success. *American Psychologist, 52*(10), 1030–1037.

Sternberg, R. J. (1997b). *Thinking styles.* New York: Cambridge University Press.

Sternberg, R. J. (1998). A balance theory of wisdom. *Review of General Psychology, 2,* 347–365.

Sternberg, R. J. (1999). Intelligence as developing expertise. *Contemporary Educational Psychology, 24,* 359–375.

Suchman, A. (2004). Toward an informal curriculum that teaches professionalism: Transforming the social environment of a medical school. *Journal of General Internal Medicine, 19*(5, Pt. 2), 501–504.

Swenssen, R. G., Hessel, S. J., & Herman, P. G. (1982). Radiograph interpretation with and without search: Visual search aids and the recognition of chest pathology. *Investigative Radiology, 16,* 145–151.

Swidey, N. (2004, March 21). The self-destruction of an MD. *Boston Globe,* pp. 20–25+.

ten Cate, O., Snell, L., Mann, K., & Vermunt, J. (2004). Orienting teaching toward the learning process. *Academic Medicine, 79*(3), 219–228.

ten Cate, T. J., & Smal, J. A. (2002). The transition of medical education from a discipline-oriented to a problem-oriented approach. In E. Van Rooij, L. Droyan Kodner, T. Tijsemus, & G. Schrijvers (Eds.), *Health and health care in the Netherlands* (pp. XXX–XXX). Maarsssen: Elsevier.

Trapnell, P., & Campbell, J. D. (1999). Private self-consciousness and the five-factor model of personality: Distinguishing rumination from reflection. *Journal of Personality and Social Psychology, 76*(2), 284–304.

Ward, M., Gruppen, L., & Regehr, G. (2002). Measuring self-assessment: Current state of the art advances. *Health Science Education, 7*, 63–80.

Wear, D., & Castellani, B. (2000). The development of professionalism: Curriculum matters. *Academic Medicine, 75*(6), 602–611.

Weaver, C. A. I., & Bryant, D. S. (1995). Monitoring of comprehension: The role of text difficulty in metamemory for narrative and expository text. *Memory and Cognition, 23*, 12–22.

Wegner, D. M. (1994). Ironic process of mental control. *Psychological Review, 101*, 34–52.

Weisman, J. & Connolly, C. (2005, August 31). Poverty rate continues to climb. *Washington Post*, AO3.

Wells, A. (1994). A multi-dimensional measure of worry: Development and preliminary validation of the Anxious Thoughts Inventory. *Anxiety, Stress and Coping, 6*, 289–299.

Wells, A. (2000). *Emotional disorders and metacognition: Innovative cognitive therapy.* Chichester: Wiley.

Wenzlaff, R. M., & Wegner, D. M. (2000). Thought suppression. *Annual Review of Psychology, 51*, 59–91.

Westberg, J., & Jason, H. (1994). Fostering learners' reflection and self-assessment. *Family Medicine, 26*(5), 278–282.

Whitehead, A. N. (1929). *The aims of education.* New York: Free Press.

Wilkinson, T. F., Challis, M., Hobma, S. O., Newble, D. I., Parboosingh, J. T., Sibbald, R. G., & Wakeford, R. (2002). The use of portfolios for assessment of the competence and performance of doctors in practice (Papers from the 10th Cambridge Conference). *Medical Education, 36*, 918–924.

Williams, W. C. (1984). *Doctor stories.* New York: New Directions.

Williams, W., Blythe, T., White, N., Li, J., Sternberg, R., & Gardner, H. (1996). *Practical intelligence for school handbook.* New York: HarperCollins.

Wilson, T. D. (2002). *Strangers to ourselves.* Cambridge, MA: Belknap Press.

Wilson, T., & Schooler, J. W. (1991). Thinking too much: Introspection can reduce the quality of preferences and decisions. *Journal of Personality and Social Psychology, 60*(2), 181–192.

Winerman, L. (2005). What we know witho ut knowing how. *APA Monitor, 36*(3), 51–52.

Witte, M. (1993, January–February). Witte's curriculum on medical ignorance. *New Physician*, 6.

Yancy, J. M. (1992). Response to letter to the editor. *American Journal of Surgery, 163*, 365.

Zajonc, R. B. (1980). Feeling and thinking: Preferences need no inferences. *American Psychologist, 35*(2), 151–175.

Zimmerman, B. (1990). Self-regulated learning and academic achievement: An overview. *Educational Psychologist, 24*(1), 3–17.

Zimmerman, B. (1995). Self regulation involves more than metacognition: A social cognitive perspective. *Educational Psychologist, 30*(4), 217–221.

Index

Pediatrics in Practice
A Health Promotion Curriculum for Child Health Professionals

Henry H. Bernstein, DO

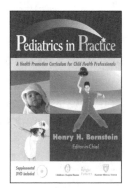

"I would recommend this book as a guiding force to exercising the privilege of serving humanity through the practice of medicine and pediatrics. The author has filled an important niche in a pediatrician's armamentarium for dealing with patients, families, and communities."

—Sanjivan V. Patel, MD, FAAP
Neonatal-Perinatal Medicine and Pediatrics, Long Island College Hospital, Brooklyn, NY

This innovative curriculum developed by the Bright Futures Health Promotion Group teaches both the core concepts and practical skills that support child health professionals in providing optimal care for children and their families.

The curriculum is based on six core concepts that serve as the foundation for effective health encounters: Partnership, Communication, Health Promotion/Illness Prevention, Time Management, Education, and Advocacy.

Partial Contents:
- Facilitator's Guide for Pediatrics in Practice
- Health: Introducing Pediatrics in Practice and Bright Futures
- Partnership: Building Effective Partnerships
- Communication: Fostering Family-Centered Communication
- Health Promotion: Promoting Health and Preventing Illness
- Time Management: Managing Time for Health Promotion
- Education: Educating Families Through Teachable Moments
- Advocacy: Advocating for Children, Families, and Communities

2003   312pp   0-8261-2175-6   hardcover

SPRINGER PUBLISHING COMPANY

The Task-Oriented Processes In Care (TOPIC) Model in Ambulatory Care (with CD-ROM)

John C. Rogers, MD, MPH
Jane E. Corboy, MD
William Y. Huang, MD
F. Marconi Monteiro, EdD

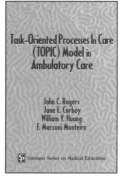

Task-Oriented Processes In Care (TOPIC) Model in Ambulatory Care

John C. Rogers
Jane E. Corboy
William Y. Huang
F. Marconi Monteiro

Springer Series on Medical Education

TOPIC (Task-Oriented Processes in Care) is a breakthrough framework of learning and teaching in ambulatory care. The TOPIC model offers guidelines for optimizing a chronic illness visit, a check-up/preventive visit, a new problem visit, a psychosocial visit, or a visit where a behavior change is recommended. The TOPIC guidelines work with any presenting problem and direct the practitioner to apply both the most current medical knowledge, and the most useful skills and approach to each visit.

The book offers instructors innovative and practical ways to teach medical students and residents how to implement the TOPIC model. The accompanying CD-ROM contains essential teaching handouts, Power Point slide sets, templates, scripts, evaluation forms, video clips, and more.

Partial Contents:

- Task-Oriented Processes In Care (TOPIC) — A Practice Model for Ambulatory Care
- Clinical Application in Ambulatory Care
- Classroom Teaching About the TOPIC Model
- Classroom Teaching of Clinical Content
- Clinical Teaching Through Supervision
- Independent Study With Cases • Faculty Development Through Preceptor Training
- Evaluation

2004　160 pp　0-8261-2425-9　hardcover

11 West 42nd Street, New York, NY 10036-8002 • Fax: 212-941-7842
Order Toll-Free: 877-687-7476 • Order On-line: www.springerpub.com